PICK AN AIRPORT...!

Entertaining and insightful stories of
a world-weary physiotherapist

by
Nathan Ohio

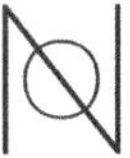

ISBN: 9798852600899

Book and Cover designed by Natalia Rykiel
Title fonts designed by Rocketpixel / Freepik

All events portrayed actually occurred, but for reasons of privacy all names, locations and timelines have been changed and obfuscated, bar one. Substantive corroborative evidence and proof of each and every episode is readily available.

First and foremost to Natalia, without whom this book would undoubtedly still be unwritten.

To Oli & Mel gor there exspurt pruff-reeding asisstunse.

To Jazzy for his grammatical guidance, innit.

To Susan for her lifelong, unwavering support and help, and Bobby for just being...

To Rosie for her unconditional affection and attention.

And lastly to all my good friends, too numerous to mention (well they're not, but who doesn't like to feel popular?!), for all the help they've provided, big and small...!

A friend, Richard, once said, "Nathan, you're a bit nuts, ...but in a good way!" When I asked him what made him think that he replied, "You've just told me that yesterday you saved some- one's life, by giving them CPR in the hospital foyer, and when I asked how you felt, all you said was, 'Very happy I'd saved 'em, but a bit pissed off that I missed my lunch break'!" So when I told Richard I was planning to write this book he just laughed and said, "Doesn't surprise me. Actually I've been reading a few like that lately, some are quite interesting, and your mad life and mental side could make yours pretty entertaining." He thought for a minute, then offered, "You should start with some sort of resume of your crazy, quirky life to date mate, it's what they all do and to be honest you'd have a pretty good story to tell. Yours has been pretty wild Nate, I mean, arts-performer, athlete, admin' assistant, bouncer, waiter, child-care officer, murder/terrorist suspect (only for two hours - an unnerving case of mistaken identity) and all the other stuff. It'd make a pretty good intro' at least, and there ain't many people with that sort of a history, especially not physiotherapists, well, not as far as I know anyway!"

"Yeh, not a bad idea", I replied. "Not sure how I'll be able to do it though, at least not without incriminating myself and a lot of other people too, you included! Never mind, maybe I'll find a way." But the more I thought about it, the less appealing it became. It smacked to me of that seemingly ever-prevalent situation on those (well-hidden) talent shows, where it's almost compulsory for every entrant to have some sort of angst and tragedy-ridden back-story, if they're ever to have any hope of getting selected. Usually one regarding their mum's friend's dog-walker's son, who, despite fighting with being severely colour-blind has donated one of his ears to a deaf dog in Finland.

Why the title? Well, when very first thinking about the possibility of writing this book, the first 'physiotherapy' story that popped into my head was in fact the situation and catalyst that first pointed me down the road to actually becoming a physio'.

* * *

There I was lying in my swag in the middle of the Australian outback, sleepily contemplating my navel fluff and enjoying the warmth and solitude, having taken some time off to go camping in a pretty remote region, with Jane, my girlfriend at the time. I was deep in thought, pondering my options in life: Up until this point I'd been a bit of a 'journeyman', having moved from job to job, as per the intro'. I was a definite 'jack of all trades, master of none'. I could drive a car, lorry or boat; ride a bicycle, motorbike and horse; swim, snorkel and scuba-dive, and had licences to do all, along with a fair few academic qualifications. But I had no actual professional vocation and possessed no officially accredited, or certified, trade qualifications and, as such, was now pondering on how to make a go of things, both job-wise and with Jane. Possibly by either staying on in Australia with her and trying to enrol on a vocational course down there, or maybe by seeing if she would be willing to come back to the UK and live 'uptop' for a bit, as I might have more study or course options open to me. Especially to train as a physiotherapist, which was the profession I'd pretty much decided upon trying for at this point.

Jane was walking back to the tent from the tree-shower we'd rigged up and, as she approached, I sensed something was slightly amiss. I asked what was wrong and definitely wasn't ready for the reply. Jane blurted out that a month or so earlier, whilst I'd been away from home for a couple of weeks, sorting out some family problems, she'd met up with an ex-boyfriend and been, as she put it, 'somewhat intimate' with him. Or, as I read it, 'ridden him like a rodeo bull'!!!

I was stunned. I stood motionless, mind racing, thoughts hitting hyper-speed as they bounced wildly around my now near-exploding head, and they went precisely as follows. "Well, that's it. Relationship's over, holiday's over, don't want to be with her another second. Can't leave her here in the middle of fucking nowhere, don't want her next to me in the truck for the four-day drive back to Sydney, need to get to an airport and offload her. Same distance to Rockhampton and Mackay, she needs to choose!" And the next words out of my mouth (after what seemed like an eternity to me, but according to Jane was less than two seconds) were, "Pick an airport!" She did.

The six-hour drive to Rockhampton was one of the quietest I've ever done. Even the truck seemed to understand the situation, as the chassis had stopped squeaking and the engine was purring far more quietly than usual. I dropped off Jane, drove back to Sydney, returned to the UK, embarked upon a physiotherapy degree course and the rest, as they say, is history. The title phrase stuck in my head for quite some time afterwards, and was often used by myself and friends as an ultimatum, meaning 'you've really reached the limit of my patience now', or 'stepped over the line' type warning. Occasionally still is.

CHAPTER 1

Philosophical waxing

For the record, I think (as is indeed the case) that the vast majority of all doctors (GPs, house officers, registrars, consultants etc.), nurses, physiotherapists, occupational therapists and health workers in general are great people. Diligent, kind, moral, skilled, expert individuals, working incredibly hard to care for their patients. I applaud every one of them, feel privileged to be amongst their number and would unequivocally encourage anyone considering training to become one of them, to forge on*. However, as with any profession, there are a (thankfully very) small minority who are poorly/under-skilled, complacent or misguided. With bad attitudes and strange beliefs towards their work, responsibilities and patients' care, the combination of which can make them, at best, professionally ineffective, and at worst, downright dangerous, occasionally even deadly. The only people worse than they, are those who harm by intent rather than ineptitude, the malevolent psychopaths, the Harold Shipman's and Beverly Allitt's of this World. An additional problem to that above is that, as with many other professions such as the police and social services, we health workers hold positions of power over our patients (clients), thereby exponentially increasing the possibility for harm to be inflicted upon them by any improperly acting practitioner. In that they (the patients) place a huge amount of trust in us, and will often unquestioningly accept and permit potentially-harmful procedures to be performed upon them, or medicines administered to them, that they would not ordinarily contemplate allowing others to do, under any other set of circumstances.

---

*However, if you're doing so with the prime goal of 'making lots of money', then personally I'd say, possibly think again. Because unless you're willing to compromise yourself in some way, you're unlikely to succeed in that endeavour. Obviously it's possible, but I'd contest not without either using (less than adequate) short patient-consultation times, cutting corners by engaging solely in quick, symptom-resolving treatments, or 'charging like a wounded bull' for consultations, none of which are generally in the best interests of the patient. There's obviously always the option of 'working yourself to an early grave', with ridiculously long hours, seeing high numbers of patients, but where's the fun in that?

Unfortunately, we physiotherapists are not exempt from having some of the above-noted type, undesirable individuals included in our number.

In my 27+ years as a practitioner I've (unfortunately) been privy to some quite damning examples of poor, negligent and, in thankfully a very few (but distinctly unsettling) number of cases, tantamount to criminal practice and behaviour by some colleagues. Including one (supposedly) relatively experienced physio' who, when presented with a medically seriously-ill patient, complaining that their tablets were 'making them feel sick', simply advised said patient to, "try stopping the medication for a few days until the sickness dies away". The only thing likely to have died in that particular scenario was the patient themselves!

Thankfully, on that particular occasion, I'd inadvertently overheard the conversation from an adjoining cubicle, was able to intercept the patient immediately after their consultation, and rectify the situation before they left the building; advising the person to continue taking their medication as prescribed and urgently seek (true) medical advice from their GP, or local hospital A&E Department. I continued on to explain to my colleague, just how professionally (and indeed criminally) negligent they had been, and the possible consequences that could have arisen from their actions - including potential loss of life, career and liberty - had the worst-case scenario occurred.

I've never shied away from addressing such matters, nor been averse to receiving 'steering advice' myself when needed, but unfortunately there are many who prefer to simply 'let things slide' and trundle along, turning a blind eye and 'hoping for the best'. It's easier, but it's not right.

To be honest, the actions of my colleague on that day were almost unforgivable. It wasn't a case of them not knowing or understanding what they were doing, but simply one of them lazily ignoring both their professional training and basic common sense.

A fundamental tenet of physiotherapy education is and has always been (to this point at least), that you never interfere in a patient's drug regimen or their medication consumption, whether it be palliative (to reduce then-occurring symptoms) or prophylactic (to prevent symptoms occurring in the first place). Including advisement on consumption of even the most basic painkillers or anti-inflammatory medications. However, more and more physiotherapists seem to be becoming increasingly inclined to ignore this dictum, especially with the advent of Advanced Physiotherapy Practitioners (APP), administering cortisone injections and feeling increasingly comfortable with the notion of medically advising patients. It's often very tempting and extremely easy to occasionally give little, quick, 'common sense', off-the-cuff types of this sort of advice to patients, especially when they request it, as is frequently the case. But the cold reality is, that any physiotherapist doing so outside of their official professional ability or remit is, as previously said, potentially risking their career, livelihood and liberty.

Real case in point. A physiotherapist had a patient who had suffered an onset of symptom episodes, whereby they were very occasionally getting inflamed wrists. The patient enquired as to whether it was ok for them to use a simple, non-prescribed, off-the-shelf type anti-inflammatory medication to help reduce their pain and swelling. Unbeknownst to the physio' being asked, that particular patient had an undisclosed, underlying mental health condition for which they were already taking medication that, as it transpires, would have reacted aggressively and very 'negatively' with the patient's intended extra medication. The physio', having given the patient 'the nod' to take said anti-inflammatory, almost ended up in a very sticky situation.

The drug in question was Ibuprofen, which reacts, often quite severely, with lithium-based drugs (causing 'lithium intoxication', a potentially life-threatening condition requiring hospitalisation) which are sometimes prescribed to patients suffering from severe &/or prolonged bouts of depression (a condition which many people are, understandably, often reluctant to divulge). Such was the case in this instance, with the physiotherapist being totally unaware of the fact.

By a stroke of luck, as they parted, the physiotherapist had quipped to the patient that they might just want to check with their pharmacist whether Ibuprofen was the best, or indeed the cheapest brand drug available. Thankfully, the patient did so, and was subsequently guided by the chemist to an alternative, safe medication. The physiotherapist only became aware of what had occurred, during the patient's next consultation and, by their own admission, 'had a mini panic-attack' at the thought of what could very easily have transpired.

My (sometimes unwelcome) response to each and every request for advice on drugs or medication from patients, and one which I'd advise any physio' (or other pharmacologically unqualified practitioner) to use, is a boringly simple mantra: "I'm really sorry, but giving you any type of advice about any sort of medication is outside my professional remit, and you'll need to ask or check with your GP or Chemist."

CHAPTER 2

Best (and most courageous) patient (I've ever had the honour to work with)

Bell

A young girl who, after having gone through more than eight hours of spinal surgery - to remove a particularly unpleasant tumour, substantial sections of bone and have titanium spinal-rods inserted - was, shortly thereafter, told that to enable further, unexpected radiotherapy treatment (to attack a residual part of the tumour, which had been deemed too dangerous to reach surgically, during the operation), she would have to undergo the whole traumatic procedure again; to remove the inserted metal rods and substitute them, with 'radiologically non-reactive' carbon-fibre replacements. Despite this ordeal, Bell remained happy, chirpy, bright, optimistic and thoroughly pleasant throughout. Bell was testament to all the best qualities of humanity (and, unbeknownst to her, the complete antithesis of another patient whom, for some unknown reason of fate, I coincidentally and repeatedly had to treat immediately after Bell). Bell's chances of survival were extremely low at the time and I lost contact with her, once she travelled elsewhere to continue her specialist treatment. However, I have it on very good authority that Bell prevailed, is alive, kicking and thriving as I write. And no doubt infecting others with her fantastic attitude to life. Hoorah!

Second best

Maude

92 years young when I had the privilege to meet and treat her. Came to the physio' department for "a bit of a push on my sore back please!" Maude had injured herself whilst bushwalking, aged 92. Yes, bushwalking! She recovered remarkably quickly, because Maude was nothing less than brilliant, displaying absolute commitment to the undertaking of any and every activity or task given her, in order to speed up her recovery and get her back walking.

Maude put many of my then much younger (30- 50 years) patients to shame. A purpose for which she inadvertently and unintentionally ended up being used for, much to her amusement. Maude would trot into the gym area full of the joys of Spring, loudly enquire as to what exercises she'd be required to perform that particular session, and then proceed to undertake them with such vigour and gusto that many of the other previously unenthusiastic patients, who up until that point had been moaning, groaning and moving with the speed of sloths on Valium, would quite literally blush with shame and feel no option, other than to lower their voices and 'lift their game'. Loved Maude, just loved her!

Two years later, I heard via a Third Party that Maude was ill in hospital, with a chest infection. It just so happened that I knew the Head of Physiotherapy at the particular hospital she was in, so I rang to ask him if he could possibly arrange a bit of 'extra-special' attention for Maude, and send her my regards to boot.

A few hours later my friend rang back and, in inimitably succinct Aussie fashion, simply said, "Sorry mate, she's pretty much cactus!". Which was his way of telling me that Maude didn't have long to live. Turned out that Maude wasn't in the actual hospital itself, but its sister hospice next door, and that her 'chest infection' was in fact multiple cancerous metastases in her lungs.

I went to visit Maude the next (Tues)day. She was still as bouncy and bubbly as ever, sitting up in bed, recounting her latest bush walk from the week prior to her admission, and explaining at length, the route she'd take on the next one, once she'd "gotten rid of this dreadful cough". Maude died that Friday. Her legacy was proof that getting older doesn't mean having to let things go!

Every person and problem has to be evaluated individually, but, that said, even so, from that point onwards, whenever I heard a seemingly self-engrossed patient with a relatively mi nor problem, bemoaning how hard it was to do their exercises, or the inconvenience it was causing them in the pursuit of 'all things trivial', I would simply think of Maude and start to compose a shopping-list in my head until the noise stopped. I once managed a whole week's worth of sundries, whilst a pampered 'Rupert' droned on, about how his still slightly bruised and swollen calf was going to 'seriously affect' his social weekend, by preventing him from wearing his favourite boots to a party. Sometimes a gun might be best…!

Worst patient

Miserable, unpleasant, sloth of a woman who, it subsequently transpired, was a serial vexatious litigator (quick 'heads-up' to all those newly qualified, 'green' physiotherapists out there, this is one category of patient that you will never ever manage to 'cure'**; at least not until they've received their pending compensation payout) They are the leeches of society and the piles to humanity's arse.

Again, please don't get me wrong. When individuals end up being negligently treated, they deserve and should receive appropriate compensation, financial or otherwise. But those who repeatedly, cynically and unjustifiably seek out financial gain, for trivial mishaps, 'non-events' or fabricated/exaggerated situations and circumstances, simply because they can (and know they will likely succeed, due to the current weakness/stance of NHS litigation-defence policies) deserve something very different. This woman was a case in point. Had a permanent expression, 'like a bulldog licking piss off a nettle', personality to match and the seemingly sole objective of complaining/litigating wherever, whenever and against whomsoever she could, irrespective of the personal, professional, vocational or financial consequences that might befall those she sullied along the way.

It quickly became obvious, as is often the case in situations such as these, that this person had initially received a completely justified financial, compensatory payout, for a genuine grievance and had then 'developed a taste' for this way of obtaining 'easy money', a bit like the mouse that keeps re-visiting the same spot in the larder where it previously found a delicious cake. As the consultation progressed, I proposed a course of treatment and management of this patient's problem, which both she and I knew would likely be very beneficial in markedly helping, if not indeed completely resolving, her problem - clinically at least - but which was different to that which she was hoping for, indeed had openly, directly requested. At this point, the woman leant forward, pointedly gestured towards her arm and whispered to me, directly, "If you don't do the treatment I want, I'll sue you and get a payout!" This person was the very embodiment of all that is wrong with people's attitude and approach towards the health service and society in general. She was pure poison and I was incensed!

Emotionally what I wanted to say isn't publishable. Professionally, what I actually said was, "I'm afraid I'm going to have to end this consultation, report and document all that you've said and re-book your appointment with another physiotherapist."

I stood up abruptly, causing the woman to flinch slightly, turned, walked the three steps to the cubicle curtain and drew it back to leave. As I pulled, I hesitated, slowly turned back towards the now slightly 'edgy' woman (who had obviously not been expecting such a response) and, scowling harshly, said very firmly, "What you've just said means that on a pure whim, you were prepared to try and fraudulently obtain some money by possibly destroying my career. I'm from a broken home, I have very little, and what I have I've had to fight 'tooth and nail' for. So just how do you honestly think I'd've reacted, if you'd done what you just threatened to?" With that I left.

I then proceeded to perform all the tasks I'd stated, along with the additional bureaucratic formalities now necessitated by such situations, and waited to see what transpired. Which was, that the woman not only failed to attend any subsequent appointments, but also dropped the (at the time unbeknown to me) multiple, ongoing litigation cases that she had concurrently running against other health professionals in the same hospital!

I believe optimum overall care of a patient should be of paramount importance and the primary function, if not indeed sole goal, of any health or medical situation and patient-practitioner interaction, I've (unfortunately) been a patient many times myself and experienced first-hand, the difference between varying levels of patient treatment. As said, where avoidable or negligent mistakes are made, patients should absolutely have the right, ability and facility to complain, be heard and seek redress. Such situations need complaints to be acknowledged, circumstances addressed, harmful procedures changed, unacceptable attitudes and work practices confronted, necessary lessons learnt and where appropriate, patients compensated, sometimes substantially so.

The flip side to this coin is that one of the current, single biggest problems, with situations regarding medical litigation, seems to be that when it comes to dubious or fraudulent patient malpractice claims, especially those of a repeat, serial nature (which seem to occur with depressing frequency these days), once it becomes known that an individual is predisposed to act in such a manner, many of those involved in their subsequent treatment become (understandably) wary and scared of them - a fear often exacerbated by poor management and lack of support from professional governing bodies. This effectively leaves the patient in control, often ensuring them a 'successful result', irrespective of the merits or otherwise of their claim. It's a case of 'the tail wagging the dog', and it's wrong!

**Others being those patients who wear their problem or pain like a 'martyr's badge', needing it as a point of reference and something of interest to talk about. Or, sadly, those who have almost 'become their problem', to the point that their lives tend to revolve around it, to the exclusion of all else.

CHAPTER 3

Best treatments

First

A gentleman from Grafton, NSW who, for reasons too lengthy and complicated to go into, I strongly suspected had bone cancer, despite his absolute dearth of signs or symptoms. As a result of which, I re-referred him to his GP and requested a check X-ray. The (understandably) somewhat reticent (due to lack of clinical evidence), but nonetheless amenable GP, arranged for said X-ray which, both unfortunately and fortunately, confirmed my suspicions.

The man was flown to Sydney two days later for an operation, which, in conjunction with a short-course follow-up of chemotherapy, saved his life. Can't really get better than that.

Second

A middle-aged man whom I saw at a large London hospital. The poor, weak and somewhat socially disadvantaged guy had very recently undergone major surgery. A 'radical scapulectomy' - which basically involved removal of pretty much his whole shoulder blade and accompanying muscles - to excise a large, cancerous tumour, which had left him with virtually no right shoulder at all. He'd been referred to the physiotherapy department for rehabilitation. As soon as the man started talking my suspicions were aroused, and after a few minutes chatting I realised the worst, the poor man's lungs were full of cancerous metastases, later confirmed on X-ray, though you didn't need a stethoscope to check. The 'death rattle' of his lungs was clearly audible from across the cubicle. It begged the question why? Why had this poor man been put through such major, very painful and obviously futile surgery only weeks before his almost certain and imminent demise?

It was Winter and a very cold one at that, yet, unusually for Britain, the sun shone almost all day every day and the hospital's rehab' gym, an old, converted, large rotunda-type conservatory, served as an immensely efficient sun-trap, making it incredibly warm and cosy, no matter how low the outside temperature.

I'd been requested to try and help the man, Paul, regain some movement and strength in his arm, but it would have been an exercise in futility. Paul had almost no muscles left in his right shoulder or upper arm, and in any case, he was generally so run-down that he really wasn't up to doing any sort of exercise. Paul was terribly weak and, on arrival for his first treatment session, actually seemed to be borderline hypothermic.

It transpired that Paul had no heating at home and little in the way of warm clothing to wear. On entering the warm, comfortable gym he promptly fell asleep on the treatment bed, basked in sunshine and with a hot cup of tea to hand - kindly supplied by the Women's Royal Voluntary Service (WRVS) volunteers. By his own admission Paul was as comfortable, warm and happy as he'd been in a very long time, chatting pleasantly between naps to whoever was nearby, and occasionally eyeing the exercise equipment that neither he (nor I) had any intention of using. I booked Paul in for his follow-up 'treatments' three times per week, every week, ensuring that each of his sessions lasted at least three or four hours, and consisted of him doing precisely the square root of fuck-all. He was happy, comfortable and at peace.

One particularly cold, wet Friday morning Paul didn't turn up for his appointment, and missed his following Monday session too. The next day I received the news I'd been expecting, Paul had died. I was happy that I'd been able to afford him some semblance of comfort before he shuffled off to the other side, and hoped he'd been warm and comfortable when he did so.

Third

One I could never have envisaged in a month of Sundays!

I'm sitting in the small, hot treatment room of a remote Australian Outback clinic when my patient walks in. She's a 34-year-old woman named Angela. A mother of two young children, who smiles pleasantly, but somewhat nervously, as she enters. She says hello and then immediately whispers, "I really don't think you can help me. It's a really big 'woman's problem' I've got and I've just been booked in for an operation at Orange Hospital in two months' time. But I'd already made this appointment before getting my op' date, so I thought I'd better keep it."

"Try me," I said, "I'm sure you won't surprise me." How wrong I was!

"Well, er, how can I say this?", she began. "Well, basically, it's like this, I've got a double, anal & vaginal prolapse and I'm doubly incontinent. It all really started after the birth of my second child."

I have to admit that for a second was more than a little taken aback and, momentarily, somewhat speechless. Though in partial mitigation for my initial surprise, it has to be said, that these were once-monthly, small clinics, which I ran in conjunction with the (magnificent) Royal Flying Doctor Service (RFDS) of Australia, in remote Australian Outback towns, and where 99.5% of my patients' problems were 'manual labour-type' injuries, usually sustained during some sort of rigorous farming or other outdoor activity.

My first thought was (somewhat patronisingly) how brave Angela was, sitting there alone in a room, explaining her very intimate and (clearly to her) acutely embarrassing problem to a male total stranger. My immediate second thought was, "Shit! Why didn't I attend those optional lectures on Women's Health all those years ago, I'm going to be about as much use as a chocolate fireguard?!" I had been certain at the time of said lectures, that they would never be of any practical help to me whatsoever, anytime in the future. Again, how wrong I was!

What transpired was an hour-long consultation, where I reached into the farthest recesses of my noggin, scrabbling around to retrieve the smallest morsels of information that might help me with my seemingly impossible quest, of, in turn, trying to help this unfortunate person. Anyone looking down on this scene would likely have repeatedly shifted, from squirming with embarrassment, to sitting in somewhat gob-smacked disbelief, as I proceeded to explain to Angela how to make anal and vaginal-sphincter strengthening, weight-training devices from tampons, watches, soup-spoons, socks and batteries'. And how to stand, sumo-style, in a swimming pool, whilst trying to suck water up her backside by repeatedly clenching her buttocks. And how to empty her bowels without straining***

The session ended. Angela stood up, thanked me and left. I knew she'd listened intently and taken onboard almost all of what I'd said throughout our session, but unhappily doubted that the exercises would be of much use to her. Or indeed that Angela would be happy/willing to perform what were, after all, quite bizarre and somewhat complex manoeuvres of her nether regions.

Due to scheduled aircraft maintenance causing a lack of transport, my next Outback clinic in that particular town wasn't until four weeks later. As I entered the reception, from the corner of my eye I spotted my first patient of the day, it was Angela, sitting comfortably, but looking somewhat 'resigned'. My heart sank! "Come in", I said, with a cheerfulness that belied my negative apprehension. "How have you been Angela?"

"Great", she replied, "everything's cleared up. I've stopped wetting myself, my bottom's fine and I've cancelled my operation. Don't know how to thank you, you've changed my life."

For the second time in as many months, I was taken aback and speechless! "A pleasure", I replied, still slightly in shock. With that Angela kissed me on the cheek and left, but not before handing over a substantial donation to the RFDS (which many people don't realise is actually a charity) and a box of chocolates for yours truly. I have seen tens of thousands of patients during my career, but to this day, these three treatments remain the best I have ever given…!

***This is an area of concern for a great many people, not just those with pre-existing problems, nor is it limited solely to a person's physical and functional aspect(s) but also their situational and psychological ones. I'm not really qualified to help deal with the latter, 'getting your head read', aspect of such matters (though I do have a few, possibly worthwhile, cursory tips), but I can give some, potentially quite helpful, advice regarding the former two factors.

As far as 'situational' is concerned. If you're averse to using public toilets for 'number twos', from an hygiene perspective, then simply always carry a small bottle of alcohol-based hand sanitiser and pack of wet wipes with you (many people now routinely do so anyway, due to habitual changes as a result of the recent Covid-19 pandemic), and use them to wipe/disinfect the toilet seat (and inner bowl-rim if desired, re. dangling appendages). Then do what many, again, already routinely do, which is put toilet paper on the seat and (again re. 'danglings') drape some over the front and down into the pan if necessary.

You can of course employ the age-old and frequently used (mainly by women) method, of hovering. However, contrary to popular belief, this isn't actually particulary helpful, bowel-clearance-wise at least, because it actually increases abdominal tension and reduces overall bodily relaxation. As regards easy and satisfactorily complete bowel emptying, if you're having problems, with continually straining and/or 'retention', then try the following technique.

Firstly, do not actually go to the loo until you really need to, regardless of whether it's the 'correct' or 'allotted' time (straying a little into 'psyche' territory here) - and by 'really need to', I mean like the times when you've had to do the arse-clenching, 'trying-not-to-shit myself' walk, 50 metres from home. Then, once seated, do not attempt to actively push or strain your bowels in any way whatsoever, but simply relax, take a deep breath in and then slowly, gently exhale through open, widely-pursed lips, as if you're 'frosting' a mirror. If nothing happens the first time (often the case) then, again, do not push or strain, but simply repeat the action and continue doing so until you feel movement in your bowel. At this point resist the very tempting urge to push now, and instead continue simply deeply breathing in and exhaling. When you feel your bowel starting to empty, don't push, but simply exhale more forcefully (but still 'smoothly'). Only push, gently, almost at the end of emptying.

It's actually possible to 'blow-empty' your bowel without pushing at all. If at any point you feel like you do need a bit more pushing, instead of using your stomach muscles, simply put your thumb in your mouth, seal your lips round it and blow, as if you're trying to inflate a balloon. Hey presto!

Close runner-ups

The 65-year-old farmer, who had had almost constant pain in both arms and not a single unbroken night's sleep for over 3 years, meaning that neither had his wife, as they still shared the same bed. He'd previously had unsuccessful treatment to both his arms and only came to see me because the pain had become so intense, that he'd suffered what's known as 'pain-inhibition' of his arm muscles, causing him to drop a lamb whilst carrying it. He was on the verge of 'retiring early', as a result of the pain and his increasing inability to work, and had come to see me pretty much as a 'last resort'.

It transpired out that the unfortunate man was simply suffering from what's generally known (by us dinosaurs) as, 'Thoracic Outlet Syndrome'. A condition whereby stiffness, pressure and irritation to the (facet) joints of the lower cervical (neck) and upper thoracic (chest) areas of the spinal column, cause general inflammation in and around the spinal joints, which in turn pressurises the adjacent nerves running through and around the area, resulting in pain and weakness in the back, shoulders and arms. It was actually an 'easy fix', which simply consisted of three treatments, over a five-week period, of gently massaging, mobilising and gently 'loosening up' the farmer's spine, after which he was completely and utterly pain-free. The man's first words on seeing me, for what was to be his fourth treatment session, were, "I've got a bone to pick with you, mate!"

"Oh shit!", I thought, "it's all gone wrong!" It turned out that the bone he wanted to pick, was that he jokingly blamed me for him having been late to work the previous day, because he'd slept in that morning, due to having had his first pain-free, deep and full night's sleep in over three years. His wife baked me a cake to say thank you, it'd been her first good night's sleep for that time too.

* * *

The businessman who had suffered crippling back pain for five years, so bad that at times it had sometimes caused him to move around his house on his hands and knees, unable to stand. Any treatment he'd received over the intervening time had simply been ineffective, or even made things worse.

I came across him by chance, treated him once (as a favour to a friend), with the most basic (but, critically, correctly selected and targeted) lumbar spine mobilisations, and immediately resolved 95 percent of his pain. The remaining five percent took a few more days to clear. This result was not because of my having any super-powers, but because over all those years and treatments the man had simply never once been fully and appropriately assessed. I was the first person to have simply taken the time to look at him properly.

This is a situation that is becoming ever more prevalent in today's NHS with patient physiotherapy consultation and treatment times dropping from 60 to 45, 30, and even 20 minutes in duration, with professional governing bodies simply standing by, allowing it to happen. Some people (elderly, infirm, disabled or otherwise) can take up to 10-15 minutes just to get themselves undressed and ready for treatment, so it doesn't take a genius to imagine what 'quality' of assessment and treatment they're likely to experience given those aforementioned time allocations.

* * *

A high-level, Eventing & Dressage (horsey go backwards, horsey go sideways…) competitive horse rider, who, similarly to the previously mentioned farmer, had suffered two years of unremitting, almost continual and intense pain down both arms, which three consultant surgeons, four physiotherapists and two osteopaths (and a partridge in a pear tree) had previously been unable to resolve. Resulting in the patient preparing to completely give up their competitive exploits, work and lifelong association with all things equestrian, due to being unable to cope with, or perform even the most basic, simple or menial of horse-associated activities, e.g. couldn't to pick up a bucket of water, lead a horse, or strap on a saddle without crippling pain in both arms.

Diagnosis and treatment was as per the aforementioned farmer, and reason for previous non-resolution of their pain was the same as for the above-mentioned businessman. End result, complete cessation of all their symptoms and return to full 'horsey' activities within eight weeks. Along with bundles of gratitude and boxes of chocolates!previous non-resolution of their pain was the same as for the above-mentioned businessman. End result, complete cessation of their pain and return to full 'horsey' activities within eight weeks and bundles of gratitude.

CHAPTER 4

Best non-treatment

The old boy was pushed into the cubicle in a wheelchair, sitting slightly awkwardly due to his pain, but with 'stiff reserve' in his posture nonetheless.

"So, tell me about your injury and back pain, what happened and when?", I said.

"Well", he replied in a very polite manner, but with clipped, 'upper-class' tone and delivery, "it all began about 55 years ago…!" My heart sank. I was still relatively new to physio' and very inexperienced, but already knew well, that this sort of extremely chronic (i.e. long-lived) pain was generally almost impossible to resolve. "There I was", he continued, "just tootling along, when all of a sudden, whoosh, bang, ratatatat!!! Bloody Gerry! Out of the sun! Sneaky blighters had blindsided us. Anyhow, we gave as good as we got but there were too many of them, and next thing I know, blam-blam-blam!!! Armour-piercing rounds are making Swiss cheese out of my engine and I'm ditching in the Channel. Boys from the lifeguard picked me up and I went back to face the music!"

It rapidly dawned on me that this man was one of 'Winston's few! An actual World War II fighter pilot, who'd helped ensure that we are as we are, and live as we live today...! Ordinarily, at this point, I would have started to try and direct the conversation back towards the clinical Q&As, but I was mesmerised and simply said, "Spitfires?"

"No", he said firmly, but gently, smiling as he lifted a halting forefinger.

"Hurricanes then?!", I retorted.

"Nope", he replied quickly, almost pre-empting my answer, still smiling and now gently shaking his head.

"Must've been Tempests then", I said, now hitting the limit of my WWII British Fighter Aircraft, pub-quiz knowledge.

"Oh good man!", he exclaimed, "most people have never heard of them. Good man!"

"Go on", I said, now completely enthralled.

"Well", he continued, "got home, got another kite and got back up there. Well, blow me down if it didn't happen again. 'Fool me once, shame on you, fool me twice...' eh!? Got really shot up this time though, much more serious, one round went straight into the back of my chair."

Now knowing that most Spitfire, Hurricane and Tempest pilot seats at that time were reinforced and armour-plating, to withstand penetrating enemy rounds, but also realising that the shock-wave of being hit by one could still seriously jolt someone's spine, regardless of whether or not it actually penetrated the seat, I said, "So is that when you hurt your back then!?"

"Oh no, no", he replied, "but as I said, things were a lot worse this time 'cause I had to bail out over occupied France. Anyhow, the French Resistance found me and spent a couple of months smuggling myself and some other chaps down south to the Pyrenees, ready to sneak over the border into neutral Spain. We got there and were just heading off to cross the border, when we were ambushed by the Germans. Bloody traitor in the ranks! Set us up, good'n'proper! Well, terrible firefight, few killed, but most of us escaped. Got a nine milli' right in the arse though, and THAT'S when my pain started young man! Been bothering me on-and-off ever since".

This fantastic man then continued to regale me with his further exploits, including flying Hurricanes (which he "preferred to Spits" because they were 'tougher' and 'beefier') and landing out of fuel, on country roads. I looked at my watch, an hour had passed in an instant. Not only were we out of time, but I'd actually overrun into my next patient's session slot by five minutes, and not written down a single word.

"Oh shit!", I thought. "I am sooo very sorry sir", I said, plaintively, to the genial hero, "I haven't done a thing with you and we're already completely out of time. I'm actually going to have to re-book you for another 'first' appointment, as I don't have time to do anything now. I really am truly sorry, I honestly don't know what to say!"

"Nonsense", he retorted briskly, "it's been a pleasure chatting to you. My pain's waited 55 years, a few more days won't hurt eh, pardon the pun."

I hurried over to the reception desk and requested that the gentleman be re-booked in asap.

"There's no free, new-patient slot for at least four weeks now, so I'm afraid he's just going to have to wait", said the somewhat stern receptionist.

I don't remember her name but do recall that she was in her 50s, quite strict (as many are, and indeed have to be), but a very fair-minded and decent woman.

"He's a bloody war hero!", I whispered to her, across the desk in frustration. "It's entirely my fault I know, I totally stuffed up and I'm sorry, but there must be something you can do?! Can't you just cancel one of this lot?", I said, gesturing with a slight flick of my head towards a couple of 'revolving door patients', who happened to be seated behind me at the time - some patients repeatedly present to physio depts, regarding treatment(s) for problems which many would consider 'trivial' and, no sooner has said problem been resolved, than they re-present with another: they're known as 'revolving doors'.

The secretary looked at me with a mixture of admonishment and understanding, narrowed her eyes, smiled like the Cheshire cat's cynical city cousin, that's just seen a blind mouse, and whispered, "Leave it with me, I'll see what I can do."

Three minutes, four rapid phone calls and one hasty conversation with the patient transport office later, 'Biggles' had his new appointment set, ...for the very next day.

I loved every moment of Biggles' company over the next few weeks, during which he regaled me with further war and flying exploits, and was absolutely delighted when, at the end of our course of sessions, we'd managed to clear almost all of his pain, save for the rare, occasional, short-lived twinge. My biggest regret was that I didn't remember his name, partly as a result of professional habit, borne of patient confidentiality, but mainly because, just like a magician, Biggles had blind-sided and engrossed me so deeply and effectively with his exploits that, to my shame, I forgot about the man himself.

CHAPTER 5

Biggest serving of 'humble pie'

It had been a looooong, long morning. I was tired, somewhat grumpy and waiting for my last patient before lunch. Twenty-five minutes past his appointment time, and therefore too late to be treated, he rushed through the waiting room door.

"Sorry!", I said, holding up a rebuffing hand and jumping in before the man had a chance to say anything, "you're way too late for your appointment, you'll have to book another one!".

"Oh, ok," replied the man, dipping his head slightly, with an (unusually) understanding resignation in his voice, as he turned to approach the receptionist's desk.

"Why were you late anyway?", I asked, somewhat gruffly, my annoyance thinly disguised as I casually started to cross the room, intent on continuing straight on to the hospital cafe, five minutes early.

"Er, well, I was here in plenty of time, but I ended up giving CPR (cardio-pulmonary resuscitation) to someone in the car park, …and that's what made me late I'm afraid," said my patient, lowering his voice as he spoke, seemingly almost embarrassed at his life-saving exploit.

"What?!", I snapped, whipping my head around, face half-frowning, a mix of part disbelief and part shock, thinking that either I'd misheard the guy or that he was royally taking the piss!

"No, it's true", chimed in one of the receptionists, a little too gleefully for my liking. "One of the A&E nurses just came in a moment ago and told me what was going on!"

"Ah, I see", I said, somewhat sheepishly, now slowly turning to face my patient. "In that case, you go on ahead to the cubicle Mr X, just give me a second and I'll be right with you!"

And with that I walked back across the foyer and reception area to pick up the man's notes from the office, casually but avidly flicking the V's to the two receptionists, who by this stage were both ducked down behind their respective desks, doubled-up in gut-wrenching pain as they tried, very unsuccessfully, not to wet themselves laughing at my current situation and obvious extreme embarrassment.

CHAPTER 6

Most heroic colleague

Rebecca was a very demure but equally chirpy person. A happily married mother of two, who, by her estimations, was average height, average size, average ability and had an average outlook on life. But that couldn't be further from the truth. Apart from her exceptional fortitude and stoicism, and being an extremely competent physio', Rebecca had a highly infectious laugh. One so forceful, that when it emanated from her throat, with the speed and impact of a tank-busting rocket, it seemed to surprise and catch her off-guard as much as it did everyone else, …every time!

Rebecca also had the memory of an elephant. So much so, that I truly felt sorry for her husband and kids, because they just couldn't get away with anything, whatsoever - "I've never, ever said that, Mum". "Yes you have. You did last April, when we were on holiday at…". I once momentarily forgot the name of a girl I'd been dating some years previously, whom I'd told Rebecca about only twice, briefly. She was not only able to instantly rattle off the girl's full name, but also precisely where she lived! I always said Rebecca should've worked for one of the intelligence services, who knows, maybe she secretly did?

Heroic because, for over a year, Rebecca carried on working, sometimes in excruciating pain (undoubtedly far greater than that of any patient she was treating at the time) whilst undergoing prolonged treatment for cancer, and told no one at work other than myself, swearing me to secrecy. She never complained, was always chirpy and just got on with life. Her attitude, outlook, and manner were a testament to all that is good with humanity and put many self-pitiers to shame, myself included.

Second most heroic colleague

Dan was a short, fit and very pleasant man, whose modest looks belied his ability, and who, as a person and practitioner, had a very idiosyncratic perspective on life. Dan's personal mantra consisted of two words, 'too weak'. An ethos which he applied to almost all aspects of life, including the rehabilitation of patients. There were very few grey areas with Dan. If someone couldn't complete a (by his standards) reasonably levelled exercise or task, then they were, in Dan's eyes, simply "Too weak mate!".

Now, some might think that this was a bit of an excessive, or even inappropriate attitude to have towards a(ny) group of patients, but Dan's clients were a very special set of individuals. All of them needed, and were highly intent upon, returning to 100% fitness asap, in order to be acceptable for their intended assignments and activities. "Too weak!", I'd hear him shout, as some man-mountain, Wednesday-man ("If he says it's Wednesday, it's Wednesday!") struggled with his 47th consecutive press-up.

"Too weak!", as an exhausted patient started to falter on the rotating, inclined, stair-climb machine; all the while smiling, and giving his clients encouraging, cheeky winks.

On rare occasions, one of Dan's clients would partially or wholly 'spit the dummy', refusing to continue or finish a task. At which point Dan would simply demure, and let them be. He never forced anyone to perform any task and, on one occasion, when a relatively young, inexperienced, thoroughly-exhausted and poorly-informed lad, tried to accuse Dan of 'giving more than he could take', Dan simply smiled and wandered off, leaving it to others to inform the young man as to just how wrong he was.

Because, not long before that day, Dan had been overseas in an active war zone and, due to combat logistical difficulties in accessing appropriate equipment and backup, had sat himself astride the landing strut of an Apache attack helicopter, totally unprotected and taking incoming enemy live-fire, whilst being flown directly into the live hot-spot of a particular battle-zone, in order to (successfully) retrieve a severely injured colleague who'd been shot. In the process, personally helping lift said wounded man, and attaching him via a sling-harness to the underside of the helicopter. Dan was one of those (increasingly rare) people who actually 'walk the walk' before they 'talk the talk'.

"Too weak!" best (carrot and) stick phrase ever, especially for lazy arses with large egos.

CHAPTER 7

Small island escapades

The small clinic had just one treatment room, but it was wonderfully large, spacious, light and airy. I was filling in at a temporary, 8-week posting and though a long way from anywhere, actually felt quite at home, having been made extremely welcome by the locals and staff, especially Edith, the chain-smoking, 'seen-it-all', perennially unfazed secretary with a highly infectious, throat-rumbling laugh.

"Come in", I shouted, and my next patient entered. To say she was the most beautiful, athletically fit woman I'd ever seen would be a lie, but she was very close. I finished the subjective, pre-assessment questioning and, as it was a lumbar spine problem she was suffering from, then requested that the woman undress down to her underwear, if she was comfortable doing so, put the two supplied towels around her chest and waist respectively and then let me know when she was ready.

"Ready!", she shouted, less than a minute later. I entered the room, froze, tried unsuccessfully to stop my jaw from dropping and then tried to compute what I was faced with. My patient was casually standing in the middle of the room, stark naked and smiling. For a nano-second or less, two equal and opposite thoughts shot through my mind; "Wow!" and "Shit!".

For the second time in my working life I impersonated Rudolph Nureyev, rapidly pirouetting on the spot, exiting the room at ultra-high speed and then, through the slightly ajar door, shouted, "Can you put your underwear back on please!"

"I don't mind!", she sang.

"No, but I do!", I replied, visualising my licence to practise floating off out of the big bay window.

"Ok, ready now", she shouted. I re-entered the room, only to repeat my previous action, but this time with a plaintive cry, under my breath, of, "Oh Jesus!".

The woman was standing in exactly the same position as previously, having dutifully put on her underwear. However, said underwear consisted solely of what could only be described as a single, postage-stamp-sized piece of mosquito netting, held in place by some strands of dental floss and, again, she was wearing no top.

"Please can you put one of the towels round you!", I once again shouted, through the crack in the door.

"I really don't mind", she warbled, "honestly I don't, and anyway the towels won't stay on me. Can we just carry on as is, it's ok, really it is".

"Shit!", I thought, "What am I going to do?!" Then the answer hit me. I'd have to get Edith the secretary, to sit in on the session. This I did, although the consultation then had to be immediately suspended for five minutes, whilst 'Smoky Joanna' had one of her innumerable fag-breaks (which were ordinarily taken whilst the physiotherapists were busy treating their patients). The session then proceeded without further event, other than Edith casting me the occasional glance and surreptitious flat-line smile, both of which said, "I know why I have to be here, but hurry up, my nicotine levels are bottoming out!". I completed my assessment of the patient, or 'Missy with the bum-floss panties', as Edith subsequently referred to her, and all was well.

Now, I don't know whether the few women's underwear shops, on that particular island, stocked exclusively 'lower-half-only, mosquito-netting' type underwear apparel but, suffice to say, that such was the regularity of similarly-repeated 'underwear episodes', I very soon ended up having to move Edith and her desk into the treatment room on a permanent basis, for the rest of my tenure. Something that went down like bacon at a bar mitzvah with my chain-smoking sidekick.

Several months later, on a cold winter's day, I was sitting in a car, bemoaning how hard I worked, whilst also relaying this and other stories to one of my best friends, Robert, a tough, hairy-arsed builder who, being quite interested in health and fitness, had asked me to explain to him the process of a physiotherapy 'standard patient assessment'. I did so and, after I'd finished, he said, "So, let me get this right, Nate. You just got to spend three months on a beautiful island, watching loads of people, often women dressed only in their underwear, waft in and out, bend up and down a few times, day-in, day-out, in a bright, warm room, with soft music playing, and you're now trying to tell me it was hard work?! Man, you don't know you're born. I'll swap you any day of the week. You can go up and down ladders, carrying bricks in the pissing rain, and I'll sit on my arse, watching the wafters. Just say the word soft-arse!" With that, he dropped his head and slowly started to shake it. He had a point.

* * *

"Doctor Nathan, Doctor Nathan, can yuh come quick, tekk a look at dis an see what yuh tink!?"

"I'm not a doctor, I'm a physio, and technically speaking not a fully qualified one for another four weeks!", I shouted down the corridor.

"Nooo, but yoo look lyke wan, an dat's goodinuff!", sang Chantal, the incredibly perky Physio' Assistant, in her strong, thick, lilting Caribbean dialect. "Enniweh come, come quick, yuh gotta see dis!" And with that Chantal headed towards the department gymnasium, vigorously beckoning for me to follow. I was on a Caribbean island, two weeks into my six-week final elective placement, at the end of my Physiotherapy course, having fortuitously been able to arrange it during the preceding year.

The hospital was clean, tidy, well-maintained and the staff were all professional and diligent, but the facilities, resources and access to necessary equipment/medicines, were all shockingly poor. At the time of my arrival, there had been six patients in the hospital's Intensive Care Unit (ICU).

Now, though I have a good understanding of 'much stuff medical', I'm not a doctor and nor would I pretend to be, despite Chantal's labelling. However, with concurrence from a number of friends, who are indeed highly-experienced medics, I can say with a fair degree of certainty, that in the UK five of those people would almost certainly have recovered, and one might have had about a '50:50' chance of survival.

When I left the island, six weeks later, five of the poor souls had died and one remained 'critical'. It was not a lack of care that did for them, far from it, it was a lack of resources and facilities. E.g. Nurses & physio's having to re-use 'single-use' suction catheters (used to clear the phlegm, sputum and mucus from the lungs of unconscious patients), multiple times on the same patient, with just a wipe-down to clean them and storage in a jar on the wall, at the head of the patient's bed, in an ambient, humid temperature of 28 degrees centigrade. Chances of contracting a secondary infection, probably 99.99%...!

"Look look! Go on man, show 'im!", encouraged Chantal, talking to the relaxed, laconic, 40-something guy who was currently leaning over, propping up the gymnasium wall.

The man dutifully complied, stood up, stretched out his arm and bent his elbow. Both Angela (a junior physio') and I observed the movement and could find nothing untoward.

"Noh, dooit again, dis time propali, all di way!" admonished Chantel.

The man sighed comically, momentarily and simultaneously raising both his eyebrows at myself and Angela, then, again, dutifully bent his elbow. Again, nothing unusual seemed to be happening.

I glanced sideways at Angela, giving her a slight shoulder shrug and half-frown, as if to say, 'what's going on?'; which she reciprocated. Then it happened! At about 90 degrees, the man's arm continued to bend, but this time the movement was occurring not at the elbow, but at his mid-forearm and markedly so! The man was rapidly forming three sides of a square with his arm.

I was transfixed, momentarily hypnotised, but then recovered and turned around, just in time to see Angela bolting towards the door. She managed to make it down the corridor and into the washroom, but unfortunately not to the sink in time, before unceremoniously dumping the contents of her morning's breakfast, all over the toilet block floor!

"Shouldn't bi soh now shud it sah?!", said Chantel, grinning triumphantly, knowing she had discovered something very unusual, which she indeed had, very much so.

"How long's it been like this?", I asked the man.

"About six months or so I guess,", he replied.

"And why didn't you come to see someone about it sooner?" I enquired, more than a little perplexed.

"Well, to be truthful, it wasn't really bothering me at first", he said, "and it wasn't bending as much as it is now. Then a few weeks ago I felt another 'pop', and then my whole arm started to bend a lot more, but it still didn't hurt. I only came because now I can't push or throw things with that arm, and I need to for work sir."

What I surmised (and in fact transpired to be the case), was that the poor guy had suffered painless, full-thickness cancerous necrosis of both his radius & ulna (forearm) bones, causing the (clinically) catastrophic event we were now observing.

The man was swiftly allocated appointments for a same-day X-ray and blood test, then, almost equally as swiftly, flown off to Miami, USA for further specialised treatment.

Chantal was quite rightly, strongly complimented and commended for her care and actions, for it was she who had insisted on bringing the man to our attention, when he'd in fact only been referred for just the simple provision of an arm brace or cast, in order for him to re-commence working. Due to his 'lack of fuss' and laconic, quiet demeanour, had Chantal not intervened, this is very likely all the care that the man would have received, with likely disastrous and fatal consequences.

I left my placement before the man returned and I never found out how he'd fared, but I hope he had the best possible outcome, in making a full recovery.

I returned to the island some years later (having established a 'twinning' of the main, island hospital with my course-study hospital in the interim period), to invigilate during examinations for a newly-established University of the West Indies, Physiotherapy training course, and once again see, one of the best bunch of staff I'd ever worked with. (C.D., E.B & V.B. et alles). Happy days!

CHAPTER 8

Reality life

One day, whilst working at a certain major teaching hospital, I had just taken a new patient into my cubicle and then subsequently left to get a form I was missing, when Sarah, a very pleasant, affable and always energetic physio', emerged from her cubicle in synchro' with me, looking slightly flustered and more than a little shocked.

"Have you got a new patient now?", she whispered.

"Yes," I replied quietly, "why?".

"Too difficult to explain now," she said gently, looking slightly distraught, "but please could you swap with me and see the guy I was supposed to, I just can't have him as my patient."

"Of course," I said, immediately starting to feel a little angry, because it seemed obvious to me that the man must have done something inappropriate to upset Sarah.

We swapped patients, and though remaining professional throughout, I have to say that I didn't exactly exude huge amounts of warmth towards my new patient. After both our sessions had ended, I went to the staffroom and asked Sarah what the problem had been. She told me, and I was, well, simply gobsmacked.

What has to be borne in mind when reading what follows, is that as well as being pleasant, affable and extremely attractive, Sarah was also a very, very reserved. A 'non-spontaneous' type of gal, who generally planned out her life and activities, sometimes down to the last detail.

At the start of the proceedings, Sarah had gone to the waiting room and called her patient's name. As he'd stood up, she had physically gulped and, as he entered the treatment area, Sarah had, in her own words, 'momentarily lost it'! She recovered, got a grip of herself, asked her patient to be seated and then to confirm his name, DOB, address, occupation and family status (all standard ID verification, pre-assessment questions). The conversation had then gone precisely as follows:

Sarah: "I'm afraid that I won't be able to carry out your assessment today, sir."

Patient (somewhat perplexed): "Oh, why not?"

Sarah (unable to believe the words emanating from her mouth, as they did so): "Because if I do, you'll officially become my patient."

Patient (now extremely perplexed): "Er, ok, so what's wrong with that then? I don't quite understand!"

Sarah (now heading gently into something close to psychological shock): "Well, that would mean that, under professional patient-practitioner guidelines, we wouldn't be able to socialise and so you then wouldn't be able to take me out for dinner, sometime, ...hopefully!"

Patient (now not sure if he's actually awake and wonders whether they were just normal mushrooms he'd eaten for dinner the night before): "Eh?!"

At this point, Sarah, having never even contemplated, never mind actually done anything even remotely like this before, went quite light-headed and actually almost fainted. She realised the potential ramifications of her actions (especially if things went the way they very easily could have at that moment), but also instinctively realised that for her, this particular guy was, as they say, 'the one!!!'

"Oh, I see!", said the man, having thankfully, rapidly grasped the situation into which he'd just been launched, as Sarah attempted to stay conscious and prevent her now fire-engine red face from hitting the floor. "Sounds good to me."

Sarah's relief was instant and incalculable! The man accepted her invitation and, as it turned out, he was indeed 'the one'. I know this because, a couple of years later, I heard on the grapevine that the two were married and expecting their first child.

I think it's fantastic. Though at this point there are likely a few 'certain types', up there in the echelons, as spontaneous as Swiss bankers, currently huffing and puffing lots of hot air about the above scenario. Quick to condemn, but faster than shit out of a goose, when invited to fully-catered, day-long meetings to discuss the nuances of KPI's, CPD, EBP or other 'vitally-important' professional and corporate acronyms, monikers or etiquettes. Yet they almost invariably do fantastic impersonations of hippos moving through treacle, whenever it comes to actually making substantive decisions, or acting substantially upon, genuinely important issues, such as (re)establishing adequate patient-consultation times, addressing the lack of equal opportunities or inordinately high levels of racial discrimination within the ranks of the physiotherapy profession, and the health sector as a whole. Still, I'm sure all the hot air they generate comes in very useful for filling the balloons at Christmas!

CHAPTER 9

Prison time - six degrees

Physiotherapists occasionally treat prisoners. Often 'on location', in the prisons themselves, but sometimes in hospital departments, for necessary care that's not available in their particular correctional facility. As a treating practitioner, it's rare that you ever get to know what offence the individuals have committed and, as a general rule best not to - unless of course, not doing so might compromise either the patient's treatment or practitioner's safety, or both - but the degree of their crime's 'severity' can often be roughly gauged, by the number of handcuffs they're wearing, number of guards escorting them and number of guns being carried by said escorts.

I'm obviously not going to say where, when or even in which country I saw this particular person, but on our first and every subsequent encounter he was escorted by 4 prison guards, 2 armed police officers and had a police helicopter buzzing over the hospital for the whole duration of each and every visit. These themselves were always a surprise, given that, for obvious security reasons, they were always organised, booked and enacted in secret, and at extremely short notice, generally less than two hours prior, having been booked into the clinic diaries under fictitious names.

Matt was an absolutely immense guy (built like a Challenger tank), extremely fit, but also very friendly and thoroughly likeable. So I was intrigued to know how someone seemingly so nice, could've ended up in his situation. I never asked, but on about our third treatment session Matt volunteered his story. He'd killed three people (with his bare hands) in a fit of sustained rage. Initially I was somewhat shocked, but once Matt had explained to me the reason why, I not only fully understood but, have to say, actually sympathised with the man. He had come home one day to discover that members of his family had been brutalised and killed, in the most appalling way, by a gang of men. Unfortunately for the perpetrators, Matt found out who they were and got to them before the police did…

...jump to seven years later. I'm on holiday. I've just stepped off a coach and am looking at a poster of upcoming events in this holiday-mecca paradise, when I feel a tap on my shoulder.

"Nathan! How are you my man?!" It was none other than Matt. He'd apparently served 21 years of his (whole-term life sentence) and had just gotten out of prison on 'permanent parole'. "This used to be my favourite holiday destination", said Matt, with a big beaming smile creasing his face. "I still know a lot of people here, so if you need anything Nathan, just let me know, anything at all. I'm staying down at ##########, come and visit any time. You were good to me Nate, really fixed me up good'n'proper, I owe you man!"

I didn't ever actually get to meet up with Matt, nor manage to take him up on his offer, but did occasionally see him from a distance, in passing, over the next two weeks and every time thought, "You really never know!"

CHAPTER 10

Past medical history

Reasons why Past Medical History (PMH) and History of Present Condition (HPC) are so vitally important (yet too often under-examined, skirted over or missed out completely). I was working at a large city hospital, when a lad in his early 20s came in for his first appointment.

He was a big, fit rugby second-row player and looked in the prime of health, but had experienced ongoing and undiminished neck pain since a clash of heads during a game some weeks earlier.

I started the 'subjective' part of my assessment, finding out all about how and when his pain had started, then, when it came to checking his past medical history, given that he was by his own admission in perfect health, was about to skip my normal detailed enquiries and simply move-on to the practical 'objective' part of the assessment, in order to save time. But, at the last moment, I decided to stick to my normal, somewhat dogmatic but professionally correct questioning routine.

It turned out to be a good move, possibly one of the best of my career. When I got to the 'gastro-intestinal' question, the lad told me that he'd previously suffered from Crohn's disease for some seven-plus years, and had been routinely taking the then standard treatment, of moderate to high level steroids such as Prednisolone, for that whole period. The steroids were part of the reason why he looked so fit and strong, having promoted extra muscle growth. However, they were also likely responsible for this young man's ligaments probably being far weaker than normal for someone of his age.

Steroids are anabolic for (build-up) muscles, but catabolic for (break-down) many other bodily tissues, especially those containing collagen, such as ligaments, tendons and bone (a lesser-known fact that many athletes would do well to be very aware of). A subsequent MRI scan of the young man's neck, showed that this was indeed the case. So significantly in fact, that the poor guy had to immediately stop playing rugby and any other contact sports, for fear of possibly suffering a severe, possibly catastrophic, permanently debilitating neck/ spinal injury.

The relevance to me was, that the problem this patient was suffering from would ordinarily have been appropriate to treat with some, generally highly effective, vertebral mobilisations. These are gradate-force movements of individual neck vertebrae, proportionate to a person's stature/physique. Given the lad's general, deceptively large build, mobilisations towards the firmer grade would have been deemed appropriate. However, had I done so, ignorant of his medical status, I could possibly have exacerbated the patient's problem or even injured him further.

* * *

A senior physio' I once shadowed at a private clinic, to professionally observe their various treatment techniques, diagnosed a patient as having Achilles tendonitis, by using a 'special scanning device' (no idea to this day what it was, possibly a Star Trek phaser). They then issued said patient with a very expensive walking boot and referred them on to a private consultant, for topical, cortisone injection treatment to their tendon.

What this practitioner had missed, or, despite their experience and expertise, failed to consider, was that the patient had a prior history of similar pain episodes in both their left and right calves and none of the symptoms had ever been triggered by any sort of traumatic event. Throw into the mix that the person worked in a very physical job and suffered frequent low-back pain as a result, and it was quite likely that at least part, if not all, of this patient's leg pains were the result of lumbar spine nerve irritation, causing 'referred pain' into their calves. A few additional, diagnostic, neurological tension tests, would certainly have helped make things a lot more more clear, but these were never performed. It's truly impossible to know for sure, but I'd be prepared to wager quite a lot, that some basic treatment to that patient's lumbar spine, together with a few stretches, postural correction exercises and gentle, sciatic nerve mobilisations would have markedly helped, if not fully resolved their problem. The patient certainly hadn't responded to prolonged and ongoing episodes of topical, symptomatic treatment, to their calves over a prolonged period, the medical equivalent of 'painting over rust' or 'changing a flickering lightbulb when the faulty wall switch is actually the problem'.

After the patient had departed I tactfully gave my thoughts, rationale and opinion to the physio', but they fell on deaf ears. To me that particular practitioner ranks right up there, with the senior, band 7, specialised spinal-expert/lead-physiotherapist I once came across, in a home counties NHS hospital, who stated to her colleagues (in all seriousness), that you didn't need a patient to take off their clothing (or indeed, even their coat) in order to perform an acceptable and accurate spinal assessment on them. Or the (again) senior physiotherapist, who couldn't see the problem with trying to perform lumbar spine traction on a patient, whilst said patient was wearing braces, with their jumper and shirt tucked into their trousers. I 'guesstimated' that about 1kg of the 20kg traction-pull was actually going through the patient's body, with the other 19 kgs doing a wonderful job of decreasing his shirt.

Every profession has them, colleagues who are about as useful and effective as a sponge in a tsunami.

* * *

'The call' went up midway through the long-haul flight. 'Bing-bong'. "If there's a doctor on board or any passenger with medical training or knowledge, could they please make themselves known to a member of the crew!"

At that point all the academic doctors (of philosophy, education, business etc.), who'd been upgraded to Business Class on the basis of their 'Dr' title, sank surreptitiously into their seats, silently groaning and closing their eyes, in the hope that when they opened them again there wouldn't be a member of the cabin crew, standing expectantly over them.

I dutifully pressed my call button. Shortly thereafter, the Cabin Services Director (CSD), head of cabin crew, arrived and said, "Thank you sir, but we're fine now. A couple of doctors are attending to the sick passenger. He seemed to be having difficulty breathing, but they're about to give him some oxygen, so hopefully he'll be ok."

I was in an aisle seat and the stricken passenger was also sitting in an aisle seat, on the opposite side, about three rows down from me, so I had a relatively good view of the somewhat fraught activities that were currently occurring around him. The two doctors looked extremely young to me, but

I initially put that observation down to my own ageing - many police officers were also starting to look inconceivably young to me at that time too. I watched all the activity with a slowly increasing sense of concern.

The stricken passenger was, to me, clearly displaying signs and symptoms of a particular condition - pink face/highly developed neck muscles/'reverse-action breathing' - that the two doctors seemed to be blissfully unaware of, at this time. Partly due to the fact that in the process of helping the poor man they were not actually 'engaging' with him.

I beckoned the CSD over and hastily explained my thoughts. He looked a little sceptical, thanked me very politely for my opinion and then said, "I think the doctors seem to have things well under control now so maybe we should leave it to them for the moment."

"Ok," I said chirpily, "hope so."

The junior doctors administered the oxygen and the man's rapid, 'choppy' breathing started to calm down nicely, but then continued to slow and eventually falter.

All of a sudden, the two doctors started to look a lot less confident, positively panicky in fact. The CSD, recognising the worryingly fast deterioration in the man's state, swiftly appeared at my shoulder. "Could you please come and help?!", he asked, in that very calm yet incredibly urgent tone that only seasoned aircraft cabin crew seem capable of.

I approached the ill passenger and asked the two doctors if they were ok with me stepping in to help, which they indeed were, with the relief of being able to abdicate 'responsibility' for the man's fast-deteriorating situation, palpable on both their faces, as they retreated back to their seats faster than a cat out of a vet's surgery.

It turned out that the two 'doctors' were in fact 2nd Year Medical Students who, to be fair, had admirably 'stepped up to the plate' (when many, appallingly in my view, don't these days) and likely wouldn't have known what to do with the information (I was about to glean) even if they'd obtained it. Their only 'fault' was possibly succumbing to the impetuousness of youth, in being a bit over-enthusiastic, over-estimating their abilities and 'jumping in with both feet, without first testing the water'.

I knelt down, removed the old boy's oxygen mask, asked the (now very drowsy) man his name and whether he suffered from any long-term ailments (PMH), specifically, Chronic Obstructive Airways Disease (COAD, now known as Chronic Obstructive Pulmonary Disease - COPD).

The man nodded and murmured, "Yes, that one, COA..." COAD is, as concisely as possible, a lung condition which affects people as follows. Normally, our bodies 'breathe automatically', because sensors in our veins & arteries detect high levels of Carbon Dioxide (CO2) in the bloodstream, triggering the lungs to exhale Carbon dioxide (CO2) and inhale Oxygen (O2).

However, due to physiological and chemical bodily changes that occur in people who've suffered from prolonged COAD over many years, they end up with permanently high levels of CO2 in their bloodstreams. In order to cope with this altered situation their bodies then adapt and begin to run on what is known as the 'hypoxic drive'. Whereby, the vein/artery sensors now react to low levels of O2 in the bloodstream, to trigger the same breathing response. So, now, if high levels of O2 are detected in the blood (for example as a result of a sufferer being given a prolonged, high dosage of pure oxygen), then the 'breathing sensors' aren't triggered, so the person doesn't breathe and lapses into unconsciousness. This was precisely what was happening to this passenger.

With his mask removed, arms braced on his meal tray to aid 'reverse-action' breathing, occasional whiffs of low- low-percentage oxygen and a little encouragement, the man's breathing slowly returned back to near 'normal'. Though it was still quite weak and shallow.

Shortly thereafter the CSD returned, with some eye-opening and very sobering words for me. "The captain wants to know what to do, it's your call."

"Sorry?!", I said, slightly startled.

"Do we turn back to Singapore or carry on to Perth? It's entirely your call!", repeated the CSD very politely.

"Ah?!?" I coughed, still playing 'mental catch-up. "As I said, your call sir," repeated the CSD. "No major rush, but currently we're about two hours closer to Singapore than Perth, and the captain wants to know as soon as possible whether we need to 'declare a medical emergency' and turn the plane back to Singapore to obtain help for this gentleman?!"

I turned to the quiet, very gentle man, asked how he felt, and whether he thought he could cope with the extra couple of hours to Australia. "Yes," he whispered, "I just want to get home, please mate." He then, very slowly, quietly and concisely, made me clearly aware that he knew he didn't have long to live ("I've got months, possibly only weeks!"), had just been to the UK in order to say (unbeknownst to them) his 'final goodbyes' to various family members and was now just heading back, to die at home in Australia.

Clinically, I should by rights have said, "turn back". But I knew that if the man was offloaded in Singapore, there was a very good chance he would never see Australia again, alive at least. I looked at the guy, thought, "fuck it, he needs to get home", then turned to the CSD and said. "Yup, he'll be fine to Perth now, he just needs some rest." Satisfied, the CSD went off to inform the pilot.

I leant forward, to my temporary travel companion and whispered, "For fuck's sake don't die on me mate, or I'll be up shit creek without a paddle!" The genial old man chuckled, squeezed my hand, winked and whispered, "Good on yuh mate". The nice old man made it comfortably home to Perth, disembarked on a stretcher, but with a big smile on his face, and we continued our flight on to Sydney.

CHAPTER 11

Blind obedience

Certain things have changed in the world of physiotherapy and not before time, for some. Most pertinent of these changes is the fact that, these days, physiotherapists are now autonomous practitioners, who make their own diagnoses, prescribe and perform their own treatments, and cannot be dictated to as such, by other medical or health practitioners. But it was not always thus.

This granting of autonomy is a relatively recent event and back in the day physiotherapists were nothing more than doctors' 'handmaidens' (back in the 1960s the profession was 99% female-populated), who could not perform any treatment unless it was prescribed to them by a GP, hospital doctor or consultant. This situation had already long changed back even when I qualified (around the same time the meteorite struck and killed all the dinosaurs), but the 'doctors are gods' mentality still prevailed very strongly with many a physio'. One such was Bellinda, a short, rotund, ill-tempered woman. She was, by all (but her own) accounts, a lazy and ineffectual Superintendent Physiotherapist, presiding over an archaic outpatient department, in which morale was so low that, on any given day, 40% of the permanent workers were off-sick and which was kept afloat by locum physiotherapists making up to 75% of its total staff numbers at any one point in time.

Bellinda hated anyone who held an opinion, medical or otherwise, that didn't concur with hers and had her head so far up the consultants' arses, that most days you could barely see her ankles.

One particular morning I went to ask Bellinda a question. A young lad, with his mother, had presented with a referral from one of the hospital's senior consultants, stating that the boy had an ankle sprain which needed treatment. However, I had assessed the young man and, even with my pitifully small, three months' qualified post-graduation experience, had been able to ascertain that the boy had in fact, very likely fractured not sprained his ankle. So, politely and gently I asked Bellinda how I should go about contacting the referring consultant, in order to relay my findings to him.

"Why do you want to speak to him?!", she demanded.

"Because I think this young boy actually has an ankle fracture," I replied.

"What did the consultant say it was?!", she retorted, almost snorting as she did so.

"A sprain," I said.

"Well then treat it as such!" she snapped, loudly.

"Well, actually I can't," I countered. "I've already written in my notes that I believe it may be a fracture, so I'll be professionally and medically remiss, as well as possibly legally liable, if I don't follow up on this. So I really do need to speak to the consultant."

Yet still, Bellinda resisted, stubbornly refusing to give me the necessary information, resulting in my having to venture into the secretary's office in order to find the consultant's contact number for myself, from the staff log. I did so. Called the consultant, explained the situation and, as he was coincidentally conducting a review clinic in the hospital at that very time, he very helpfully asked if the boy and his mother would be able to come straight down to see him, immediately. I checked, they could, so off they went.

Some hours later a message came over the archaic department's equally antiquated tannoy system (imagine Butlin's without the laughs)."Nathan, telephone call. Mr X, consultant is on the line for you, regarding your patient from this morning."

I headed to the office and by the time I'd arrived Bellinda was already there, hovering like a griffin vulture. I picked up the receiver, listened for a moment, expressed my gratitude and solemnly hung up.

"Well!!??!!", demanded Bellinda, triumphantly, legs astride, hands on extremely wide hips, glaring like a psychopathic raccoon and almost snarling. "What did he say?!"

"He said it was indeed a fracture and thanked me for discovering it," I replied, calmly, enjoying every syllable of my ego-deflating sentence, and using all my worldly self-control to refrain from adding, "So go fuck yourself!"

Bellinda was devastated. Not since Margaret Thatcher got deposed by her own cabinet have I ever seen someone so full of their own importance deflate so rapidly. It was like watching the Hindenburg go down and, I have to say, a joy to behold. Bellinda never spoke to me again over the next five months I was there. Joy!

* * *

On a slight segue, at that same hospital another locum physio', Kev, who, unbeknownst to me at the time, was to become a lifelong friend, was working in the Neuro-Rehab gym with a young lad who'd become paraplegic, after a tragic car accident and was, quite understandably, very depressed.

The young guy happened to be into bobsleighing and so, one day, in an attempt to perk him up a bit, I decided to do a surprise Skeleton-rider impersonation for him by running and balancing on my stomach atop a small, but very fast-rolling, wheeled stool. I had opened both double doors at either end of the large rehabilitation gym, in preparation for my stunt and, once Kev and her (long story) patient were positioned on the wide Bobath treatment plinth, I took a long run-up from way down the corridor, launched myself prone on the stool, and whizzed, prostrate through the gym.

Imagine my surprise when, as I sped through, I saw not only Kev and the lad, who both saw me, but also the backs of three of the hospital's board of governors who'd paid a surprise visit, to come over and observe how the Neurological Rehabilitation Department ran. I just kept on rolling by and, to this day, those three individuals have no idea as to the reason why both Kev and her patient fell over, and nearly off the plinth, laughing uncontrollably and unable to speak! More importantly, the episode helped lift the young lad' spirits, temporarily at least.

CHAPTER 12

Secret behind the smile

Dave was quite simply a great guy, with an infectiously soft, giggling type laugh, an all-accommodating helpful personality, a brain the size of a planet (Einstein/genius-level in fact) and a warm, friendly, almost permanent smile.

I usually say that you should rarely trust a person with no enemies, because, generally, they're either too wet to hold their own opinions, too 'politically expedient' to ever reveal their true selves, or too weasely and obsequious to ever say anything other than whatever they think the person they're talking to wants to hear. There are however exceptions. Totally nice, likeable people, with whom no one can find fault, because there are none.

Dave was one of those exceptions. Everyone loved him and no one had a bad word to say about him. But Dave had a deep, dark secret, one that he'd shared with nobody for most of his life. As a child Dave had been brutally abused by his father, and the mental effect it had on him proved to be catastrophic. Unbeknown to all but a few, Dave almost continuously wrestled with his inner demons, frequently secretly drinking himself into oblivion, and regularly crying himself to sleep at night. There are thousands of lifetimes of research and evidence on this subject, but a very simplistic 'street' view is simply this, the bigger the brain the more to damage, and Dave had a very big brain. One day Dave got up, got dressed, got a rope and took his own life. Never assume that smiling means happy...

Never assume

I arrived early, as always, on my first day at a new posting and walked into the department reception area, where Clare, the head physio' was awaiting my arrival. Clare didn't hide the fact that she was genuinely pleased to see me, a pleasant change from my previous placement, where I'd been greeted by the senior physio' as if I'd walked in with shit on my shoes and immediately requested coffee and cakes.

Clare quickly proceeded to show me round the department and commence the obligatory, departmental, pre-work induction course. "We have a sort of 'hot desk' policy here," said Clare, as we entered the physio' office, where all clinical notes were written, filed and appointment schedules logged. "So no one has an assigned desk as such, but whichever you pick first thing in the morning is generally yours for the day, unless there are more physiotherapists than desks and computers, in which case you might have to share. Anyhow, as you're first here go and set yourself up, I'll come and run you through the log-on procedures and things shortly."

I walked to the farthest corner, tactfully selected what I assumed would be the least desired desk-space, being as it was the darkest one, with no window outlook, hung my coat on the chair back (contravening health & safety rules) and proceeded to commence turning on the computer.

"Erm, I think you might be on my computer," said a gentle voice, very quietly and politely, from directly behind me.

"Oh?!", I replied, a bit confused, assuming that someone was possibly just casually getting a bit 'hierarchical' with 'the new temp' guy' (as sometimes happens).

Having been told only minutes before that this wasn't the case, I said, "I'm sorry, but I was told only a moment ago that I could choose any of the desks to work at," I replied gently.

"Yes, ...except that one, that one's mine, honestly it is," said the voice, even more sweetly.

"Oh yeh, why's that then?", I enquired in a mock, gently jokingly-accusatory voice, having discerned the person behind me was actually someone very pleasant. Smiling, I turned to my right and tilted my head back to see who it was trying to 'commandeer' my desk. As I did so, the person behind me simultaneously bent down to my left, to pick something up off the floor, and so all I saw was her back. As I began to turn to my left to see who I was talking to, I momentarily noticed that the computer screen had come on and that there was something wrong, as it had a lot of 'fuzzy, dead pixels'.

"Think the screen's broken," I said, as I continued turning to my left, attempting to synchronise my movement with and see, the bobbing Muhammed Ali impersonator behind me, who had now just proceeded to bob to her right.

As I turned for the third time, to my right, I felt something cold, wet and rather unpleasant push into my left hand, which at this point was dangling down beside the chair. I simultaneously whipped my hand away and swung my head around further.

"Hi, I'm Julie, this is Hanna and that's my computer," she said gently, "only because it's configured to my needs and probably not really much use to you, or anyone else really, though you're welcome to try and use it if you want. I'm game if you are!?"

We both laughed and Hanna waited patiently for me to move out of her way, thereby unblocking access to her rug which I'd just that moment noticed under the desk. The fuzzy dead pixels were highly magnified letters, and Hanna was a beautiful guide dog.

CHAPTER 13

Corrupt practice

I've come across many 'Belinda types' in positions of authority within the physiotherapy world over the years, many simply passively and (thankfully) benignly ineffectual, but unfortunately some less so.

One example was that of Nigel, the head of physiotherapy at a large city hospital, whom I'd gone to have a discussion with about a situation that had occurred the previous evening. It eventuated that a young, male, junior physiotherapist had been booked a new patient as their last consultation of the day and, despite having a full complement of staff (I was locuming there, temporarily, to cover a maternity-leave position), due to a combination of poor diary rostering, senior management negligence and the fact that the whole department was a complete and utter shambles, said junior was going to be the sole physiotherapist, in fact sole person, left alone in the department, other than the patient themselves. The nearest other member of staff was a receptionist, who was physically some

20-25 metres away, via two sets of solid, swing-type, soundproof corridor fire-doors.

Furthermore, it transpired, that the scheduled patient was female, strictly religious, had actually previously, verbally requested a 'female-only' physiotherapist at the time of booking her appointment and was to be accompanied by her special-needs child.

It was a potential 'recipe for disaster' and, once aware of it, I had no option other than to stay on in a monitoring and observational, colleague-accompaniment role. When I explained this to the boss, his casual reply left me stunned. "Oh, happened again, has it? I'll have a word with Pam in a bit."

"Again?!", I said, realising by his delivery that Nigel meant this situation had occurred, not once, but multiple times before. "Are you serious?! That's a potential powder keg waiting to explode, man. Not my problem, my post finishes in ten days' time, but if I were you I'd get on the case!"

Nigel shrugged, with all the effort of someone who simply didn't care. I turned, walked away and 'that was that'. It subsequently transpired, sometime later, that Nigel really didn't care. The reason was the same as to why the whole department was 'up the cock'.

It was revealed that Nigel's almost permanent physical absence from, and lack of hands-on input to, the department, was because, for years, he'd been running his own, very lucrative, private physiotherapy clinic, from his NHS physiotherapy office, …during his NHS working time!!

Nigel's activities eventually came to the attention of hospital top management, who investigated and subsequently drop-kicked Nigel out of the service and NHS to boot. But he seemingly managed to dodge having to front up to the Physiotherapy Tribunal Board.

Personally I think Nigel should've been prosecuted, or at the very least made to refund his NHS pay for the time of tenure during his dual private clinic/NHS roles. No idea what he's up to now, but going by current events, he'd probably make a great MP!

CHAPTER 14

Ignorance is bliss

He was clueless and she was carefree. We think he might have been brought up in a Dutch monastery, or on a remote island by Jesuit priests. 'Cloggy' was a clean-cut, good-looking lad, fresh out of physio' school in Holland and an all-round nice guy. But to say that he was a little naive, would be akin to saying that Einstein was a little bit clever.

His patient of note at the time, was an attractive girl who basically 'fancied the pants off Cloggy', figuratively and literally, and was, by her own admission (to the appointments secretary), "as horny as a rhino". By our group estimations, she also had the emotional stability of a chimp on crack. A veritable 'critical incident' waiting to happen. The moans, groans and sighs that emanated from the cubicle, whenever Cloggy was treating this patient, were so loud, startling and 'obvious', that every other patient in the department (including in the waiting room, so piercing was the hollering) went quiet, either in abject shock, or unbridled enjoyment at the soundtrack to which they were currently being subjected. Every single physio' started talking very, very loudly and demonstratively, in vain attempts to either cancel out the noise or distract their patient's attention from it. But in good old British style no one said a word about what was occurring, other than one elderly lady who, with a highly entertained grin on her face, chuckled and exclaimed, "Ooh I say!"

On this particular day, Cloggy left the cubicle to allow the girl to dress and walked into the small Physio' Outpatient's office - where the rest of us were already casually waiting, having all somewhat conveniently managed to finish treating our respective patients a minute or two earlier. He closed the door, took off his 'Clark Kent/Superman' glasses and said, in all seriousness and with a heavy Dutch accent, "I really don't understand. She only has a slight, mid-thigh muscle strain and gluteus muscle knot problem, and I'm massaging them both very gently, but she still seems to be in a lot of pain. Also, this was her third treatment in two weeks (those were the days) and she's not getting any better. She asked me to push a bit harder on her gluteus strain, but I was too worried that I might hurt her some more!"

It was all we (seven) could do to keep some semblance of straight faces. I could see tears welling up in Kev's eyes, Deb had the beginnings of a suppressed-laugh snot-bubble forming, at the edge of her left nostril, and at least two others had to 'exit stage left' at a rate of knots, in order to get far enough away for Cloggy not to hear them breakdown into bouts of uncontrollable laughter!

Karen, the Physio'-in-Charge at the time, realised that she had to step in and act fast, in order to prevent Cloggy, and possibly the whole department, ending up as headline news in some national tabloid paper or on a local tv current affairs programme.

By the time it came for Cloggy to approach reception with his patient and book her a follow-up appointment, he was perplexed to find that his whole diary for the following six weeks was completely booked up, jammed solid in fact, with new-patient referrals and follow-up appointments, and not a spare slot in sight. Meaning that his patient had to be allocated to a different physiotherapist for her next treatment. Interestingly, once the alternative arrangements were in place, the young girl made a miraculously fast and full recovery, after only one subsequent treatment session with her replacement (female) physio'.

CHAPTER 15

Sleepy time

Neurological Physiotherapists are often some of the most intuitive, skilled and downright patient people in the world of physiotherapy. Academically, I find this area of physiotherapy and medicine fascinating, but clinically, it puts me to sleep, every time. Well at least the hands-on, rehabilitation treatment aspect does. I truly love it, but unfortunately there's something about the generally ultra-calm atmosphere, warm settings and slow, gentle rhythm of the treatment sessions that I find irresistibly soporific. So much so, that it often had me snoring like an elephant seal, within minutes of starting any treatments. I'm even nodding off now, just thinking about it.

When I did my Neuro' placement, whilst studying to become a physiotherapist, I regularly used to dream of making great improvements with the patients, helping them regain their finite hand motor-skills or gross ability to walk, only to be quietly but firmly awakened, by the surreptitious poking of my tutor's finger into my thigh, with them staring at me intently as

I awoke behind (and thankfully out of eyeshot of) my patients, struggling to re-open my eyes having once again dozed-off.

During one such placement, I was paired with a lad whom we'd all ingeniously nick-named 'Dougie' (after Dougie Howser, the child-prodigy, tv-show doctor, on account of the fact that he looked about 12 years old), and we were on a ward that truly, was the 'saddest' in the hospital, in that it was the one on which all the patients have sustained severe head injuries and are markedly, neurologically compromised, being unable to care for themselves in any way and, tragically, often likely to stay so for the rest of their lives. However, though 'saddest' by nature of situation, this particular ward was one of the brightest in the hospital, with a warm, friendly, caring atmosphere and staff that would lift even the lowest soul.

Dougie and I had been given the task of helping a man who had sustained a severe head injury from a motorbike accident, which had caused his whole body to go into what is known as 'general flexor spasm'. A situation whereby the main large flexor muscles of the body are over-stimulated and stay very tight, causing the body to go into a cramped, foetal-type posture. If the injured person's limbs and affected joints are not routinely and frequently taken out of this hard-held position, by being manually moved, mobilised and extended, then the posture can become fixed and permanent. This in turn can cause great pain to the patient, and major problems with their daily care and hygiene. Due to the heightened sensitivity of their nervous systems, these patients are often highly reactive to various types of bodily touch and physical stimuli, a situation that can be a help as well as a hinderance. Help, because if the muscles physically 'touched' or stimulated by the therapists are solely the 'extensor groups', then they can be assist in 'opening-up' and improving the patient's posture. However, it takes a high degree of skilled handling and experience, learned over a long period of time, to do so effectively.

Dougie and I started to gently mobilise our patient, attempting to gradually extend him. We enthusiastically but carefully employed all the specialised holds, stretch techniques and movement patterns that we'd been taught in lectures, keen to try and help the man, but acutely aware that our chances of success were very low. Especially as this particular patient had experienced what is sometimes known as a very 'dense' episode; i.e. his degree of brain injury was extremely severe. Just over two hours later,

Dougie and I sat back, somewhat amazed at our success. The man lay comfortably in front of us, completely extended. It was an extremely difficult and very satisfactory result for even seasoned, skilled practitioners to achieve, never mind two inexperienced, second-year physio' students. We were understandably proud and pretty full of our- selves, keen to let our supervisor the Senior Physiotherapist and Neuro' Team Lead

- who at this point was standing at the far end of the ward - know what we'd achieved.

Dougie stood up, ready to walk over and alert our boss. As he did so, the tail of his clinical coat very gently brushed the sole of the patient's bare foot. The reaction was as fast as it was depressing. By the time Dougie had reached our supervisor, totally unaware of the reaction he'd just triggered, and she had walked over to observe the fruits of our labours, the man had returned back to his same pre-treatment 'foetal' posture of two hours earlier.

After allowing us sufficient time to wallow in our disappointment, our supervisor put us out of our misery, by explaining that the reaction we'd observed was an oft-repeated one and, indeed, the very reason why efforts like ours were vital to perform on a daily basis.

CHAPTER 16

Bedside manner

Most physiotherapists, doctors and a surprising number of consultants (for they, amongst medical workers, are the group more renowned than any other for 'abruptness') are in fact very adept at delivering news to their patients in a gentle, understanding and appropriate manner.

I've witnessed a physiotherapist explain (despite the fact that it wasn't actually her job to do so, but the situation required it) to a patient that the nature of their injury was such that there was a chance they might not walk again.

A generally accepted rule is that one should never definitively state that any particular goal or status will occur or be achieved, especially initially, because, firstly, none of us are divine beings, gods or truly clairvoyant, and therefore, regardless, can never truly be 100% sure of our assertions, predictions or diagnoses and; secondly, you can potentially destroy any and all hope a person might hold. The aforementioned physio' delivered their news so honestly, yet gently, that the person receiving it actually left the consultation feeling better than when they'd arrived, despite the nature of information they'd received. I also observed a consultant explain very gently and at great length, to a deceased patient's family, why it was that they weren't going to be able to bury their loved one within the 24-hour timeframe dictated by their religion, such that they left upset, but understanding and grateful for the respect he'd shown.

I've also seen the opposite side, a consultant, obviously a fan of 'megaphone diplomacy', who, whilst standing right next to the bed of a very ill, extremely obese woman in an hospital High Dependancy Unit (HDU) asked (in one of the loudest voices I've ever heard in any medical facility), "HAS ANYONE TOLD THIS WOMAN THAT SHE IS MORBIDLY OBESE?! THAT MEANS IF SHE DOESN'T LOSE WEIGHT VERY SOON SHE WILL PROBABLY DIE!"

One very young, but extremely brave Junior House Officer (given the strict medical, hierarchical structures and 'pecking-orders' that still exist within hospitals), sensitised to the look of fear and worry on the patient's face, stepped forward and whispered, "Well she didn't, and we were going tell her later today, but I think she already knows now!" At which point, 'Mr Megaphone' gave the 'insubordinate' doctor a deathly 'how dare you' stare, and marched on to the next bed, leaving the nursing staff to pick up the psychological pieces.

There's a time, a place and a way...

...though admittedly, sometimes that way can be difficult to find.

I remember a physio' called Jason. In his late thirties, a very friendly, affable, decent guy and a highly competent practitioner, but he had only one method of communicating with patients, that of being bluntly direct, regardless of the nature or content of information being delivered.

Jason was oblivious to the upset he sometimes unintentionally caused his patients with his forthright manner, despite having been informed of the problem with his approach on numerous occasions. There was a definite "glitch in the matrix that no one seemed able to fix, and some queried whether he might be 'on the spectrum', so seemingly inured was he to the emotions of others. Jason was from a military background, air force, and it was apparently this, along with his somewhat matter-of-fact natural disposition, that made him sometimes rather abrupt (though never harsh or unfriendly) with his patients.

I was asked if I could possibly enlighten Jason as to the 'error of his ways' and agreed to try. But alas, to no avail. No matter how hard I tried (and boy did I try) to explain, he just couldn't see it.

On my second-to-last day at that hospital, I was chatting with Jason - about the ongoing rivalry between RAF and Navy pilots and the difference between capabilities of the then, RAF

Jaguar fighter aircraft and Navy Harrier Jump-Jets - when it suddenly hit me.

"Jason! Y'know how in an emergency, if a Martin-Baker ejector seat punched a pilot out of the cockpit in one, single, big explosive hit, the necessary tremendous, acceleration force generated in doing so, would almost certainly compress their spine and cripple or possibly even kill them?"

"Yes." "And y'know how in order to overcome this problem, Martin-Baker designed the seat so there are two, smaller, 'below-critical', non-lethal, accelerative-force explosions, set off in quick succession, that still achieve the goal of getting the chair and pilot out unharmed?"

"Yes."

"Well, you need to take an ejector-seat approach with your patients mate, and give 'em two, or even three, smaller chunks of 'non-crippling' information over a slightly longer period of a time."

He got it!

CHAPTER 17

Capers Downunder

Approximately 80% of Australia's population lives within 50 miles of its coast and, given that the island continent and country is bigger than the UK and whole of Europe combined, that leaves a helluva lot of space for the other 20% to inhabit.

I once drove eight hours, non-stop, straight (not to be recommended) from Sydney to Ballina, and then looked at a map to check my progress (to my eventual destination of Cooktown, Far North Queensland). I became momentarily depressed when I saw just how little of the total distance I had covered. Take a look at a map of the country, then you'll understand, it's bloody HUGE!

To give another example of Australia's size and the remoteness of many '20-percenters' lives, I once worked for a few weeks as a casual hand on a large cattle station in the Calvert Hills, Mac-Alister Range of the Northern Territory. The terrain was unforgiving, the work was long and hard, and some of the daily occurrences were (to me) eye-opening to say the least. One day, we saw a huge crocodile pull a full-grown, grazing cow off a riverbank and drown it - I was amazed, ...no one else batted an eyelid. The permanent crew of (male and female) station workers there were hardy, tough and thought nothing of just 'popping up the road', 200 miles to Darwin, for a drink on a Friday night.

One weekend they made the 3000 mile, yes 3000, round-trip (on bone-rattling, dirt roads) to Cairns for a weekend birthday celebration - they left at 5pm Thursday, drove through the night, arrived 7pm Friday evening, partied almost continuously until the early hours of Sunday morning (with a brief Saturday afternoon siesta in a communal hotel room), left Cairns around 3am Sunday and were back to start work, rounding-up & branding, at 5am Monday morning. I kid you not!

* * *

For these 20-percenters, the Royal Flying Doctor Service of Australia (RFDS) provides a vital lifeline of medical support. As well as the urgent and emergency air ambulance service, the RFDS also routinely flies various professionals from all areas of medical/health expertise, out to provide health clinics and treatments to those living well outside the big city/town 'comfort zones'. It's very fulfilling work for all involved and at times can be quite adventurous. This includes the flights themselves, which are generally taken in a variety of small turboprop, five to twelve seater aircraft, and are not always 'plain sailing'.

In the four-year period of my tenure, as a part-time 'Outback physio', I was involved in two emergency landings and one emergency Return To Base (RTB). During one of the emergency landings, the plane's wheels wouldn't lock down, so we had to divert from the small, Bankstown airfield, on the outskirts of Sydney (where most of the Sydney-based RFDS flights departed from) to Sydney's main, Kingsford Smith airport, with a full 'blues'n'twos' emergency vehicle turnout. Everyone, including the control tower staff and pilot, expected the undercarriage to collapse on touchdown and we were all braced for impact, but the pilot landed with the delicacy of a mosquito, touching down, unnoticed, on a blind man's nose, and all was well.

* * *

"Mornin' mate!" quipped Graham chirpily, happy to see me once again grab the co-pilot's seat - the RFDS is the only commercial airline in Australia, allowed to use the co-pilot seat as an extra passenger seat, in order to maximise medical worker provision.

Happy, I liked to think, in part because he relished my (obviously scintillating) company, but in reality, happy mainly because, he'd already spotted Dr Mike's name on the passenger manifest, and was simply glad that I'd prevented said doc' from getting up-front. Dr M. was an absolute small plane fanatic and, being allowed up into the co-pilot's seat was, to him, like letting a kid loose in a sweet shop. He simply couldn't contain himself, no matter how often he was rebuked, by both pilot and passengers alike, for repeatedly wanting to touch the controls and continually leaning across, trying to talk to the pilot mid-flight - whenever he did manage to get in the cockpit, he was never allowed to use the headphones. Dr M. used to drive Graham mad! I, on the other hand (unusually for me), used to say very little, speaking only when spoken to and generally letting the pilots get on with their business of safely flying the plane.

Initial conversations between Graham and I usually started the same, before we actually took off: "So are you going to give me a go landing the plane at Lightening Ridge this time then?"

"Yes, of course mate, and afterwards we'll go on an elephant ride out to see the beaches."

"Thought so. Can't wait for the day when there's an elephant waiting by the runway."

"Ok, we're cleared to go. Speak again when we've cleared Sydney airspace." And off we'd go.

Our conversations were usually short but pretty wide-ranging, interesting and sometimes quite animated, though generally always calm and relaxed, albeit at a somewhat elevated volume level, to combat the pretty loud noise of the plane's two turbo-prop engines. Most trips were relatively uneventful.

Apart that is, from the two occasions, when they weren't and when I, very loudly, shouted 'fuck me!'

Once when, during a remote airfield takeoff, a big red kangaroo tried to jump over the plane, and landed in the propeller. "Fuck me!!!", I exclaimed, for the first time. It did not end well for Skippy, nor for the plane. Because the poor 'roo's demise caused the propeller to stop dead, which in turn caused the plane to drop below its stalling speed and drop out of the sky like an anvil. Thankfully, the plane was only about five metres up in the air and still had its wheels down, so the drop/crash wasn't enough to injure anybody. It was, however, enough to seriously damage the aircraft, give everyone onboard a severe jolt and, dramatically, set off the aircraft's Search-And-Rescue (SAR) beacon. The response to that was a (comforting) joy to behold. Within an hour, it felt like every helicopter, fixed-wing aircraft and vehicle with a High-Frequency (HF) radio in the state, was over or next to the aircraft.

Another time, we were about 20 minutes out of Sydney in heavy, low-lying fog and cloud. I was sitting in the co-pilot's seat, again, much to Graham's pleasure, when he looked across at me with what can only be described as extreme consternation on his face.

"What's up?" I asked.

He pointed at the instrumentation panel. I looked and momentarily failed to grasp what he was indicating, then I looked again and felt a shot of icy chill shoot down my back and right into my arse as it dawned on me, hit me like a sledgehammer in fact, that all the instrument needles were lying flat on their sides and all the panel lights were out.

"Fuck me!", I exclaimed, for the second time!

"My thoughts exactly," shouted Graham, loudly but calmly. "This is serious. We're flying blind!" With that he reached down to grab the independent, battery-powered, emergency radio-phone.

It wasn't what Graham said, but the look on his face that bothered me. He was one of the calmest most unflappable people I knew, an ex-Royal Australian Air Force (RAAF) fighter pilot, with nerves of steel, yet he looked genuinely worried.

"Tell them to buckle up, NOW!", he shouted, gesturing towards those in the back. I did so and, recognising the urgency of my bellowing, all nine of the specialist healthcare professionals (nurses, doctors and surgeons) immediately obeyed.

Seconds later, Graham pulled one of the most sudden and radical manoeuvres I've ever experienced in a plane. Still talking rapidly into the emergency phone, he yanked on the joystick and in less than half a second we were on our sides, one wing pointing directly up to the heavens and the other down to the ground. He then started to take us in a tight circle which, he continued for some considerable time. We were in a very busy flight path and, because of the prevailing fog, we and all other aircraft were operating on Instrument Flight Rules (IFR), which meant using the plane's radar, instruments and radio to locate and communicate with both the control tower and any other aircraft in our vicinity. But none of our equipment was working, so we couldn't do this or electronically 'see' anyone else and were therefore, effectively 'flying blind', both figuratively and literally. The emergency procedure in this situation is to contain the stricken plane to a strictly delineated, confined area and then ban all other aircraft from entering said area, which was precisely what was occurring.

After a minute or so of level circling, Graham then proceeded to slowly corkscrew the plane downwards. This manoeuvre continued for what seemed an eternity, with everyone in the back either squashed against a window or hanging by their seatbelt. You could tell Graham was an ex-RAAF pilot (many RFDS pilots are) by the fact that he was genuinely, completely relaxed and, though he tried to hide it, was actually thoroughly enjoying himself. I have to admit, so was I, having the time of my life in fact. So much so that it was all I could do to not burst out laughing. But I actually couldn't stop myself from chuckling when I looked back, to see all of my colleagues sitting wide-eyed, with 'deer-in-the-headlights' type expressions and doing their respective best impersonations of very pale granite statues. We eventually emerged from the clouds. The altimeter wasn't working, but Graham had been being fed a constant altitude-countdown by the control tower operators, so he/we knew we were at a safe height. Even so, when we actually emerged from the cloud, we were over a car park and so low, that it felt like if I'd reached out of a window I could've grabbed a car aerial! Graham instantly flipped the plane back to the (much-preferred) horizontal mode of travel, causing a couple of bumps in the back, and we proceeded safely back to the airfield under (what were now) Visual Flight Rules (VFR), to land uneventfully and well-armed for the next few months' dinner conversations.

It transpired that three weeks earlier, the same plane had been heavily struck by a lightning bolt - enough to burn a chunk out of one of its propeller blades - and, though having been thoroughly checked afterwards, had seemingly sustained some hidden and obviously undiscovered damage to its electrical wiring system. A veritable 'slow-release time bomb'. Still, all's well that ends well.

* * *

There are many very interesting characters amongst the good staff that fly out to serve with the RFDS. Claire, a GP from the Blue Mountains, was one of the loveliest and funniest. Heart of gold, but mad as a box of frogs. She was a bubbly, blond, chuckling, brilliantly talented GP, who always came back from the remote (and we're talking 'edge-of-the-Simpson-desert' remote) properties and households she visited, with entertaining stories, having had all manner of adventures and escapades on her trips. However, one in particular stands out.

We were in an Outback town, relaxing at the end of a long day, when a police four-wheel drive vehicle pulled up and out jumped Claire, closely followed by a young lamb! She grinned sheepishly (intended...), thanked the officers for the lift and then proceeded to tell us her story.

It turned out that Claire had arrived at a remote farm during the lambing season and, as she'd walked up to the porch, had noticed a single tiny lamb, corralled on its own in a small pen.

"Why is that one on its own?", she'd enquired of the farmer.

"Mother's rejected it," he'd replied, "so we'll leave it there 'til tomorrow then we'll have to knock it."

"Knock it?" repeated Claire, confused. "What does that mean?"

"Knock it on the head, y'know, kill it," answered the farmer.

At which point, Claire burst into floods of tears, picked up the doomed little creature and, holding it tightly to her body, cried, "No! You can't do that, pleeeaaase, I'll buy it off you. How much is it?!"

"Geez, if it means that much to yuh, yuh can 'ave it!" said the farmer.

So that afternoon Claire had set off on the 120km drive back to town, with her newborn lamb sitting peacefully on the passenger seat of the car and not a clue what she was going to do with it. The reason for the police involvement was simply that, halfway back Claire had firstly got bogged (vehicle wheels stuck in soft earth), for quite a long period and, shortly after having managed to extricate herself, had subsequently suffered a puncture, meaning that she had run a long way over her scheduled time of return back to town. So the clinic had alerted the police, who'd then driven out and found Claire, along with lamby-the-lamb. The officers kindly ferried both back to town, leaving a couple of their officers to complete the wheel change and return Claire's car back to the clinic, later that evening.

We were all highly amused by the story and asked Claire what she now intended to do with the little creature. It transpired that she was going to take the lamb back home to Sydney, to live on her mother's large property on the outskirts of the Blue Mountains. However, Claire and everyone else soon realised that she was now faced with a bit of a dilemma, as she couldn't return with the lamb on the RFDS plane the next day, because unrestrained animals are strictly forbidden on any such flights. Unfortunately, the same animal ban applied to the public bus service, and nobody knew of anyone local intending to make the 10 hour/700km drive back to Sydney anytime soon. Claire was well and truly stuck. Then, Graham the pilot had an idea. Two long phone calls later and it was all arranged.

The next day Claire found herself leaving town in the cab of timber haulage truck, with a big, friendly driver called Davo. Claire sitting happily in the passenger seat, with the lamb riding shotgun between them.

On our next trip out-back Claire regaled us with the whole story of events during the trip home, which was as amusing as it was (extremely) long. One of the funniest concerned the High Frequency (HF) radio comments that Claire and Davo started receiving within minutes of them starting the journey. The Aussie trucking community is so HF-linked, that drivers from all over the country can talk to each other as they travel. A driver in Darwin can chat with one in Melbourne and so on. It doesn't take much imagination to guess the types of comments that emanated from that radio over the next 12 hours. Many are unprintable, but one that made both Claire and Davo chuckle was, "Ay, Davo, I 'ear you've got a sheila and a sheep in yer cab. Bet yuh don' know which one you'd want to kiss first, ay?!"

CHAPTER 18

Hygiene

I have to admit I'm a bit of a hygiene buff. Not quite a 'freak', but possibly getting there. Though I don't think that's necessarily such a bad thing for a health practitioner. I'm not an OCD hand-washer or suchlike, I actually like a bit of unkempt untidiness, just so long as the things strewn around are clean and the floors and chairs are too, however I'm a stickler for personal, professional and work hygiene/cleanliness standards.

It pains me to have to write, that I have worked in departments where there has been only one hand-wash basin, and one hand sanitiser, servicing eight (8) treatment cubicles, and where some clinicians have regularly used the same treatment towel on numerous successive patients (sometimes all of them) for a whole day. So you can possibly understand my consternation at the time the following event occurred.

"Whoah, you forgot to wash your hands man." I couldn't help myself. It was a reflex reaction, borne of combined shock, disgust and at least a modicum of anger! The man momentarily faltered in his step, turned to shoot me a 'who the bloody hell do you think you're talking to' type of look, and continued his journey towards the door.

"WASH YOUR BLOODY HANDS!!!" I shouted angrily. I was in the toilets of a large teaching hospital, standing at the urinal doing as nature dictates, when a man had emerged from 'trap two' (who, from the odour as I'd entered, had definitely been 'dropping off the kids'). My anger was at this person's lack of the most basic levels of hygiene, my shock and absolute disgust were at the fact that, the man in question was a consultant orthopaedic surgeon!

What then transpired almost beggars' belief. The consultant stopped, turned and approached me, his face a picture of pure hatred and venom. He looked down, purposefully at my ID lanyard and then back up at me with an expression that even 'Blind Harry' could've read a mile off. I pre-empted his next, inevitable utterance. I lifted my lanyard, thrust it towards his face and said, "Mate, you're shit out of luck. You've got no power over me. I'm a Locum, …and you're a fucking disgrace, now wash your fucking hands before I report you to Health and Safety and hospital management!!!" I was a bit surprised by my own vehemency, which was more a result of this man's reaction(s) than his original action.

The consultant looked somewhat stunned, but then, amazingly, and like some sort of dutiful automaton, did as I'd requested and actually washed his hands. The fact that this man subsequently didn't know where the hand towel dispenser was (this being the closest staff toilet facility to his particular department), simply added a level of despair to the anger I was already experiencing.

The consultant then headed to the door and left, still somewhat robot-like in his demeanour. I followed him out shortly thereafter, taking time as I went, to say a little prayer asking that he never be the on-duty doctor were I ever to need any emergency surgery in that particular hospital, at any particular point in time, …ever!

One would hope that this appallingly low level of personal hygiene in anyone, never mind a frontline healthcare professional, is an extremely rare occurrence and I do honestly believe that that is so. Although I do recall the case of one surgeon (thankfully now retired), who was secretly nicknamed 'Poo- Hands' (kid you not) by his team, due to the incredibly high rate of post-surgical wound infections in many of his patients. Yes, we all know that surgeons and theatre staff hygienically 'scrub up' before every operation and wear sterile gowns and rubber gloves etc. But there are two questions that need to be considered; a) if your level of general personal hygiene is so low, then how sanitary and efficient are your hand-washing and/or aseptic donning of sterile surgical clothing techniques going to be, and, b) given that most consultants are 'gods in their own domains', which, if any, of their team members is going to be brave enough to challenge their action(s), even if they do notice something amiss?

Coincidentally at the time of writing this piece, the Care Quality Commission (CQC) were considering actually closing down the Maternity Unit at the William Harvey Hospital in Kent, after discovering '…extremely grim hygiene conditions…', which included '...doctors, consultants and other medical staff failing to wash their hands between patients, or adequately so before medical procedures'.

[I once briefly worked at that hospital, many moons ago and I left after precisely one week, for exactly those reasons!]

CHAPTER 19

Food for thought - thinking outside the box

One patient I once saw in Sydney, Australia, was a full-time house cleaner and mother, who had presented with lower back pain. An unwelcome result of having had to frequently bend over for prolonged periods of time, whilst cleaning many houses over many years. Her pain was almost continual whilst working, which, given that she regularly did 12-hour days, meant she was in discomfort for most of her waking life. The pain increased dramatically whenever the patient cleaned any baths, simply because, being so small (she was indeed tiny, sparrow-sized in fact), she had to stretch out a comparatively very long way in order to properly wash their far-side walls. Even using one hand to brace herself on the opposite side of the baths didn't help reduce her pain.

Unfortunately, 'Sparrow' also worked in a 'posh' part of Sydney, where many of the houses are very big and (unusually for Australia) have as many baths as showers, and she cleaned three to four houses per day.

After a few treatment sessions and (gratifyingly) diligent performance of a home exercise programme by Sparrow, over the next few weeks we had made good progress, in managing to almost totally clear all her long-standing pain. Almost that was, except for the onsets she invariably still experienced when leaning over, whilst cleaning those blessed baths.

We tried experimenting, with Sparrow changing her normal cleaning position, by kneeling down and bracing her chest against the side of the baths, to support herself whilst reaching across to their far sides. But Sparrow was so small, she could hardly see over the side of the baths, never mind reach their opposite sides.

Sparrow's 'bath pain' persisted, and I was at a loss as to how to help her, other than to advise that she stop working as a (bath) cleaner. It is the advice most physiotherapists are loathed to provide - 'you'll have to consider changing your job, otherwise there's a possibility that your problem and pain could become both intractable and irreversible' - but in some cases is not only highly appropriate, but actually vital for the patient's long-term wellbeing. It was at that point I had an (extremely rare) epiphany!

"Sparrow. Why don't you just climb into the baths and sit down to clean them, you're small enough!?" I said. "You could either take off your shoes, or simply put plastic 'shoe-bags' over them."

Sparrow did so. It worked! Her residual, slight pain completely cleared. So, if anyone in a 'posher' part of Sydney, who employs a small house cleaner, wonders why their 'idiosyncratic' tiny worker always locks the doors whilst cleaning the bathroom(s), now you know.

Now, at the start of her treatment Sparrow, being aware of the fact that she was moderately overweight and slowly getting heavier, had asked me to try and help her shed a few pounds. I'd explained that specific, detailed and/or extensive dietary advice was not really my remit and that, in any case, I had a very basic approach to 'dieting' - eat less, lose weight, simple - but agreed to help where I could, with some general advice.

During our first session, I had asked Sparrow to write down a record of absolutely everything that she ate and drank, every day for a week. She did, and honestly too, not missing out any morsel she'd consumed. I then took a look at the list to see if I could spot any obvious clues as to why she was putting on weight. I couldn't. If anything, this lady was taking in about 250 calories a day, too few to even maintain her bodyweight, never mind increase it! It was perplexing and frustrating for both of us because over the two-month course of her treatment sessions, despite shedding her pain, Sparrow had continued to put on weight.

At our final treatment and check session, Sparrow's daughter was present, having come along because the two of them were going off shopping together immediately after the appointment. Sparrow thanked me for having successfully cleared her pain and I explained how happy I was that I'd been able to do so, but also sorry at not having been able to help her lose weight.

"Are you sure you've written down absolutely everything you've been eating every day on that list Sparrow?" I enquired, "because I honestly can't understand why you're not losing weight."

"Yes," replied Sparrow, "honestly, see for yourself." With that she pulled the list out of her pocket and handed it to me.

"Could I have a look?", asked the daughter, politely. With nodded agreement from her mother, I handed the list to the daughter.

Sparrow's daughter scrutinised the crumpled piece of A4 paper for a few moments, furrowed her brow, laughed quietly and then exclaimed extremely loudly, "MUUUM, WHAT ABOUT THE FOUR LARGE MARS BARS YOU EAT EVERY DAY?! You haven't written those down, have you!?"

It transpired, that every time she went to clean a house, the first thing Sparrow would do was go to the kitchen, get a plate, place an extra-large Mars Bar on it and proceed to cut it into wafer-thin slices. She would then eat one of these thin slices, as a little treat and 'pick-me-up', each time she returned to the kitchen/central-hub of each house, as she went along through her day. Because this action was automatic, unconscious and an integral part of her work process, and because they were so thin as to be individually, 'consciously-negligible', eating the slices of Mars Bar hadn't registered in Sparrow's consciousness! We've all done it, eaten a packet of crisps, or sweets, or chocolates, over the course of a film/game/programme and not realised it; but the Mars Bars Sparrow was eating were, of themselves, accounting for more than 150% of Sparrow's necessary daily calorie intake!

With the problem identified, it didn't take Sparrow long to start shedding the weight and, a few months after discharge, she dropped by one day to show me how much she'd lost. It was a lot.

CHAPTER 20

Desert ships

I was at a point in my life where I was feeling I needed a change. Not in the somewhat muppetty-fluffhead, 'head thrown back', 'back of hand against brow', "woe is me" type of way, nor the need to 'find myself ' - 'there's a mirror in the bathroom' - just in an 'I'm getting stale here, wonder what else I could do and where else I could go' sort of head-space. Somewhat serendipitously, at precisely that time, I had been invited over to visit a couple of friends, Graham & Sharon, in Broome, WA, for a bit of a combined 'circuit-breaker', holiday and possible job-search.

I'd visited them once before on a holiday trip when I was living in the UK, but that time I flew in, directly from Perth. I remember the year well, it was 1997 and 'Spycatcher', a book by Peter Wright, former deputy director of Britain's MI5, had just been published in Australia after having been banned 'up-top' by the then British Prime Minister, Margaret Thatcher. The premise of the book was that a former head of MI5, Sir

Roger Hollis, was in fact a Russian mole and double agent. One of the Blunt, Burgess, Philby and Maclean cohort. Understandably, Maggie wasn't too chuffed with Peter's actions and tried to have him prosecuted Downunder, but didn't succeed. Her failure was due, in large part, to the fact that Peter employed the services of a brilliant young lawyer, who managed to defeat 'the Establishment' and secure a historic win for Mr Wright. That lawyer's name was Malcolm Turnbull, the same Malcolm Turnbull who went on to become Prime Minister of Australia a few years ago and, coincidentally, my Australian MP (Waverley, NSW) for a while when I was living there.

But I digress. I decided to take G & S up on their offer, but this time I thought I'd have a bit of an adventure getting there, by driving, via Broken Hill, Whyalla, Alice Springs and the Tanami Desert.

So, there I was, on the Tanami Track, middle of the desert, tootling along in my 75 series Toyota Landcruiser Troopcarrier (Troopie to aficionados), when BANG, I hit it! A full-grown, male camel. There are now more camels in Australia than in Saudi Arabia, and three of these 'ships of the desert' had just run out in front of me, having seemingly been playing a game of 'hide & seek' behind the only oasis-type clump of track-side trees for quite literally tens of miles. Both the poor creature's back legs snapped and all half a tonne (500+kg) of its body dropped onto the bonnet of my Troopie, momentarily lifting the back wheels off the ground. The weight and force of the camel's body cracked one of my truck batteries and disconnected the second, severing the power to my satellite phone and HF/ UHF radios in one fell swoop.

I'd had no chance of missing the poor creature. There was nowhere to swerve (hitting the track-edge soft sand, at even 50 mph, would've meant an instant rollover and a possible death sentence for yours truly) and, even though I was braking, the truck was still gliding on the smooth 'bulldust' sand that I had, unfortunately (for the camel), also just hit at that precise moment. The only thing that stopped 500kg of camel from coming through my windscreen at 40mph (and thereby saved my life) was the truck's huge, incredibly strong front bull-bar, made of old railway tracks, and its equally substantial, full-length roof rack, which projected out level with the bull-bar. The two were joined & bolted bolted together, by three upright, heavy-duty steel pipes.

So there I was, stranded, with a dead truck on the bend of a remote desert track, a severely injured camel beside me and rapidly fading light, as nightfall approached. Ordinarily, the latter fact would be relatively inconsequential, however there was another aspect to the story. About an hour prior to the incident, I had come upon the tail-end of a three-vehicle, road-train truck convoy heading to supply the Dead Bullock Soak Gold Mine, situated quite literally in the middle of nowhere.

Now these monster trucks kick up a blinding plume of dust, that tails for up to 500 blinding metres behind them and is so thick, it is impossible to see or pass them. The only way to get past them is if & when they actually, completely stop. Which is precisely what they very obligingly did, once I'd contacted the drivers over the UHF radio. I'd left them 'far' behind, but these same monster trucks would be coming around that bend in about 30 minutes, by which time it would be dark, my truck would be in the middle of the one-vehicle wide lane with no lights and it would take these massive vehicles about 400m to stop on the loose sand, once they'd actually seen my truck and the camel. A disaster was in the making!

I jumped out of the truck, heart pounding and checked the camel. The poor beast was immobile, but thrashing its long neck around violently, rolling its head and groaning loudly, obviously terribly injured, in horrible pain and sadly, in need of putting out of its misery. I needed to try and warn the on-coming trucks of the situation. The scene would become an absolute disaster if they didn't stop in time, but with both radios dead I had no way of contacting them. I grabbed my emergency torch, with intermittent-flash facility, and fluorescent warning-triangle, ran about 300m back down the track, set them up as a warning, hoping (but pretty confident) that the lead lorry driver would see them in time. I then ran back to my truck and jumped in. Thankfully was still ticking over, having not stalled during the accident, meaning I could move it out of the immediate danger zone. Hallelujah!!! I drove it about a hundred meters further down the track, stopped it, engine still running, grabbed my bush knife and then sprinted back to set about deciding how to kill the poor camel.

I firmly gripped my bush knife, timed my jump to coincide with the swinging movement of the camel's thrashing head, jumped onto its neck and started to try and slit its throat. The animal sensed my intention and powerfully flicked its head tossing me a long way into the sand and causing me to drop my knife. It was dusk, the knife was dull-bladed and camouflaged, I couldn't find it (note to self)! Time was limited, becoming more so by the second and things were now getting urgent!

I ran back up to the back of the truck, grabbed my large axe, ran back, lined up the camel's neck and struck! I was astounded, the axe actually bounced off the camel's neck as if I'd hit a tyre! I tried again, and again, twice more, but each time the same result! My axe was sharp, the cutting edge properly prepared, but the camel's thick hair was acting as an incredibly efficient protective 'axe-barrier'. I couldn't be sure of landing a direct hit on the camel's skull, as by now, understandably, it really was thrashing about, very quickly and violently. At this moment I started to experience a feeling that had been relatively alien to me up until this point in my life, one of extreme nervousness and slight panic. I had visions of the trucks rounding the bend and making a huge camel pie as they possibly hit the side of it (on the edge of the track).

One last attempt. I ran back to my truck, grabbed some strong rope, ran up the camel's back, onto its neck, avoiding its head and hard, stumpy horns, managed to loop and tie the rope around its neck, inserted the axe handle and started to turn, …and turn ...and turn. The camel's breathing slowed, it stopped thrashing and then 'SNAP'!

"Great!", I thought (in both huge relief and great sadness), "I've broken its neck, it's dead and out of its misery". Then the rope went slack, ..and the camel started to stir. I hadn't broken the poor animal's neck, I'd broken the rope! I was out of time. I had about five minutes before the convoy arrived. The camel was on the edge of the track and easily avoidable, but my truck was not and I had to get it well down the track, away from the danger zone, in case the trucks missed or ignored my warning signal, otherwise it could be toast! I couldn't pull off the track at all, because at this point its edges consisted of ultra-soft sand and bulldust, and my fully laden, fully fuelled (now) 4000kg truck would've got bogged in an instant. Nor could I risk trying a three-point turn to head back up the track to warn the truckers, because the track was quite narrow and, again, if I got stuck, side-on to the incoming monsters, in the pitch black it would be 'hello heaven' time. I pointlessly apologised to the camel, jumped in my truck and continued along the track, confident that my warning light and triangle would be enough to warn the truckers - you don't often come across track-side flashing warning lights in the middle of remote deserts, so when you do, you tend to take heed of them!

I knew there was a trackside, firm-ground stopping-off place, frequently used by desert travellers, somewhere nearby, as I'd mapped it out and had intended taking a break there in my original travel schedule and, 15 minutes later, I came across it and pulled off the track.

I must've looked a bit of a sight to the two couples already camped-out at the site, as they ate their dinner beside the log fire. My truck hood was smashed-in, the extended roof rack was mangled (but remarkably, had prevented the windscreen from getting hit or breaking) and, unbeknownst to me, I was covered in camel blood, all over my face and now not-so-white t-shirt - seems my knife was pretty sharp after all, just not sharp enough.

"Wot 'appened tuh yooz mate?!" enquired one of the guys, whose name was Bruce (truly), in one of the broadest (and at that point, most comforting) Aussie accents as I have ever heard.

"Hit a camel" I said, deflated.

"A CAMEL?!? Fuuuk mate, yor lucky to be alive, dead-set!"

"Guess so," I said.

"Is it dead?!"

"No."

"D'yuh wanna kill it?!"

"Yeh, why, you got a gun?" - I already knew the answer to that one.

We waited for the road train to pass, they'd obviously seen my warning sign and avoided the camel. Then, we set off back down the track to find the poor camel. It was pitch black, no moon and the poor creature was lying still, pinpointed and ultra-highlighted in the truck's strong spotlights.

Bruce walked up to the camel and pointed his high-powered rifle at its head. It was an eerie scene, completely silent, then BANG!!! The retort from the high-powered, long barrel was truly deafening! You'd have thought it would be the opposite out there in the vast expanse, but no, it was as if the shroud of darkness had formed some sort of acoustic bubble and echo chamber. The otoliths in my ears literally rattled. All four of the camel's legs shot out instantaneously, violently and simultaneously, forming an almost perfect cross, as if it was some sort of bizarre bouncy castle, that had suddenly been over-inflated, Then, slowly, it 'deflated' and 'crumpled'.

Bruce slowly walked back to the truck and climbed in and we both just sat there in silence.

"Breaks yer 'eart dunnit", he said very quietly.

"Yes," I replied, "it does."

We collected my warning light, still happily flashing its

'beware dead camel' message, drove on until we found a suitable turning spot, where the track and scrub were hard and level enough to do so without getting bogged, turned, headed back to the camp and, on return, sat down around the fire for a badly needed drink and chat.

I belatedly discovered that the 'six degrees of separation' rule really does apply, no matter where in the world you happen to be.**** The next day I spent most of the morning fixing-up the truck as best I could, watched the local council truck with bobcat (to move the camel fully off the track) on the back go by - news travels fast in the outback, often faster than in the city - and then continued to Halls Creek, where I 'officially reported' the camel incident, that they of course already knew about. It's testament to the strength of Toyota Landcruiser 'Troopies', that everyone I came across who heard my story said, unsolicitedly, that they believed had I been in any other type of 4wd vehicle, I'd now be dead.

I eventually got to Broome - passing the Wolf Creek meteorite crater (scene of the infamous murders and subsequent film) along the way - and had a great time there, but it wasn't for me, not long-term at least. I eventually headed off and pretty-much circumnavigated Australia in making my way back to Sydney. Some of the things I experienced along the way were almost unbelievable, for all sorts of reasons, but too numerous and long to convey here. Maybe another book for another day…?!

Six degrees of separation - again

****When I got home, a few friends and acquaintances were initially a little sceptical about my camel story (understandably so, I guess), especially as I was travelling alone at that time with nobody to corroborate my version of events. But shortly afterwards, by bizarre coincidental connection, it was unsolicitedly and independently verified for me.

As it happened Bruce (he of the high-powered rifle) and Mary lived in a place called Yeppoon, Queensland, and Mary's best friend up there, was none other than the mother of my best friend's wife, living in Sydney. I first heard about this, when I rang my best friend in Sydney a few weeks after returning from the trip, to give him a bit of travel news and ended up being told my own travel-adventure story back to me, by him instead. As said, Outback news travels fast!

CHAPTER 21

African angel

Pikk was a locum physio', working in the same department I, at a large Midland's hospital. She was one of the nicest people you could wish to meet, sweet as sugar (without being saccharin) and pleasant as pie, but never obsequious. She was kind and gentle too, but had a well-rounded, inner strength.

Pikk's only 'fault', as such, was that sometimes, her lack of 'force' in whatever she was saying or general reticence to display any annoyance she might be feeling, meant that some people misunderstood her, whilst others simply tried to 'take advantage' of her.

The latter situation was the case with a certain locum consultant and medical specialist, whom we had the misfortune to have foisted upon us, in sharing our four-bedroomed hospital accommodation flat for a number of weeks. Said specialist took an instant shine to Pikk, the very first time he saw her, as she and I sat chatting, watching early-evening tv in the flat's communal lounge. Within a very short space of time, it became patently obvious that this man had designs on being more than simply platonic with Pikk. Obvious, because whenever he looked at her - which was 99% of the time he was within viewing distance (and thought he wasn't himself being observed) - he did so with all the finesse and repugnance of Jimmy Savile viewing a schoolgirls' netball match. I swear I once saw him actually slightly salivate, when Pikk came into the lounge wearing a pair of lycra shorts!

Now, there's nothing wrong with a man fancying a woman, but, depending on your morality, there sometimes comes a point where the related behaviour becomes rather unpalatable and, indeed, completely unacceptable. For me it's when, as was the case, the man is in his mid-60s, married, with a 25-year-old daughter (3 years older than Pikk), and makes the object of his desires incredibly uncomfortable with his presence, actions and demeanour.

Pikk was very aware of 'Jimmy's proclivity towards her and attempted to make it clear she had no amorous interest in him whatsoever, but that just seemed to spur Jimmy on, In fact, things got so bad that at one point Pikk felt she couldn't enter the kitchen/lounge complex unless accompanied by at least one of the two other flat occupants (myself and a lady named Grace), for fear of being accosted in some way by Jimmy. A highly unsatisfactory situation, but one which Pikk and I dealt with relatively easily. Pikk would enter the flat most evenings after work and go straight to her room, then wait for me to knock on her door signalling that I was heading into the lounge - we were working the same hours and had similar after-work social movements, so the arrangement worked pretty well for the most part, much to Jimmy's obvious frustration and annoyance

On the rare occasions when I wasn't around, Pikk would simply either do a 'smash & grab' type meal prep', in and out of the kitchen in a flash, and eat in her room, or wait until she heard Grace enter the lounge. This was simple to recognise, because Grace's presence was easily detectable by her almost continuous singing and loud humming. Usually gospel songs, but always something loud and joyous. Grace was a very nice, kind, 'God-fearing' 'big momma' of a Nigerian woman. A chemist, who was very jovial and eternally happy, but someone whom you knew not to mess with. Jimmy knew it, and Pikk knew he did, so she knew she was always safe in Grace's presence. Though throughout this period, Grace remained blissfully unaware of the prevailing 'Jimmy situation".

All was well until the time came when I was to be absent for a week. I was heading off to help some aspiring young athletes, at a training camp. I was genuinely worried for Pikk's well-being, a situation that was as uncomfortable as it was just plain wrong. It was time to recruit Grace. I caught-up with Grace one evening, shortly before I was due to leave, and fully apprised her of the 'Jimmy' situation, watching her face become more and more concerned, then stern, and finally angry, as I progressed with my explanation, which I may or may not have slightly embellished or gilded a little, here and there. By the time I'd finished my soliloquy, Grace's demeanour was that of a Praetorian guard, tasked with the sole responsibility of protecting baby Caesar.

After chatting with Grace, I had to go and finish my packing. I headed for the lounge door, to leave. As I pulled it open, I turned and, with just a tiny touch of the Machiavelli, said, "By the way Grace, d'you know what. I'm sure I saw Jimmy stealing a pair of Pikk's knickers from the laundry a couple of weeks ago!". Grace's face turned to thunder and she looked like she'd just seen the cat crap on her Sunday dinner. Pikk was safe!!!

CHAPTER 22

Traction bedtime stories

Some years ago traction was used a lot in physiotherapy, often as part-treatment for spinal problems, in conjunction with specifically targeted exercises, and often with great success, though (as always) much of its efficacy depended upon the skill, knowledge and application of the treating practitioner (see previous 'belt & braces').

Then along came the 'clinically proven' and 'evidence-based practice' brigade, espousing their 'no definitive indication of medical benefit' or 'no acceptable clinical evidence or proof' rhetoric, and usage dropped dramatically. It seems that physiotherapy is no more immune to trends and 'tampering' than any other profession, medical or otherwise. Just as a broad comment on the latter, 'acceptable clinical evidence…' line, it's worth noting that;

a) 'clinical evidence' includes practitioner first-hand experience', otherwise known as 'anecdotal treatment experience', which in a court of law is known by another name, 'eye-witness evidence', and, b) to date, not a single physiotherapy treatment has ever been 'clinically proven' to work or be effective (the benchmark of proof is very high). Anyhoo, I digress.

So, there she was, merrily tootling along the motorway on her way home, when Ann, Superintendent MSK Physiotherapist, almost caused the mother of all pile-ups!

"SHIT!!!", she screamed, reactively, quite literally, stamping on her car's brake pedal, whilst travelling at 70mph in the motorway fast lane. "SHIT, SHIT, SHIIIIIIIT!!!"

Then, a split-second later, realising exactly where she was and the imminent danger she was now in, with her currently, rapidly decelerating car and fast-approaching van, that she could see in her rearview mirror, bearing down at a potentially life-ending rate, she floored the accelerator and raced-on ahead, quickly swerving over to the hard shoulder as fast as she safely could.

Ann sat there for quite a few minutes, cold, sweaty, shaking and panicky. "Oh fuck, oh fuck. How could I have forgotten him?!", she screamed to herself. Ann was about 10 miles from the hospital where she worked, halfway home on a dark winter's evening, having just realised that she had locked up and left the department for the night ...with a patient still firmly strapped to the traction bed!!!

Ann calmed herself down enough to be able to start driving again, pulled off the hard shoulder, left the motorway at the first exit, doubled back and then broke almost every traffic law known, getting back to the hospital as fast as humanly possible, all the while rehearsing in her head the plea she would make, to the hospital bosses and her professional governing body, in order not to be summarily sacked and struck off.

Ann arrived back at the hospital. The physiotherapy department was ominously dark and quiet, with the door locked firmly shut. Ann began to panic. It seemed obvious to her, that the patient had got himself off the bed, shouted and banged until someone had come to his aid and then left. But not before having made a substantial complaint, which would surely be presented to her (along with a P45) by the head of personnel next morning.

Anne checked that no one was watching, unlocked the door, quietly entered the department and, in the gloomy dark, peered towards the hidden alcoved treatment cubicle in the far corner of the room, where the traction bed was situated. She walked slowly and nervously towards the cubicle, physically shaking as she went and, as she neared, heard the distinct sound of snoring, and heavy snoring at that. Peaking carefully and quietly through the drawn curtains Ann saw the man, her patient, still in position, strapped into the harness, attached to the traction bed and off in the Land of Nod.

Now, apart from being a brilliant, if somewhat of an occasionally forgetful, physio', Anne was also one of the most quick-witted people I've ever known - faster on the take than Usain Bolt in a relay with a tailwind - the sort of person you always want on your side during one of those infernal, corporate, problem-solving 'team building exercises'.

Ann turned around, rapidly strode back to the front door and, in one deft move, turned on all the department lights.

"Wakey-wakey, Mr X!", she cried, "what on Earth do you think you're playing at? C'mon, up you get, everybody else has left, you're the last one. You forgot to press your 'alert button' to let us know you'd finished and you're very lucky we didn't just leave you here for the night!"

"Urgh, urgh, sorry, sorry!", said Mr X, groggily, "I must've fallen asleep."

"Yes, well, c'mon, hurry up and get dressed," said Ann, primly, in her best school ma'am voice, "we both need to get home and I can't lock up 'til you're out of here. Don't worry about making your next appointment now, there's no time and in any case all the computers are off, we'll call you tomorrow and book one then."

And with that, the unsuspecting fellow obediently and quickly dressed himself, donned his coat and rapidly left, none the wiser as to the true nature of the situation, but probably somewhat befuddled as to how and why he'd just lost two hours of his life.

* * *

It was a small country hospital, situated in a pleasantly quiet corner of the Home Counties. An area with a veritable abundance of landed gentry, hereditary Lords & Ladies and people with triple-barrelled surnames, many madder than the proverbial March hare.

"Reeeeaaaadyyyyyy!!!", she cried from behind the curtain. I ambled over to correctly position Lady C. - a real, titled 'Lady' and old dowager, of around 75 years of age - on the bed for another episode of very gentle lumbar traction, which was proving very effective in resolving her lumbar spine problem.

"Aaaggghhh!!!", I cried, trying vainly to stifle the sound, even as it emanated from my shocked mouth and as I simultaneously span around, at a speed that made me momentarily dizzy, exiting the cubicle at Mach 2! "Janet, Janet!", I cried loudly, to the assistant who was down at the other end of the long treatment area, "please, come here quickly!"

I beckoned to Janet, waving my arms to try and impress the urgency of my request. Janet quickly came over, looking, rightly, slightly put out, as she'd been halfway through helping another old, somewhat infirm patient put their shoes back on after a treatment session.

"What's up?", she said, a tiny bit agitated, but immediately mellowing on seeing the plaintive expression on my face.

"Can you please, please tell Lady Barking-Mad in there, to sort herself out. She's gone completely off the reservation with this one, and it's an image I'm never going to be able to scrub from my mind!"

Jane entered the cubicle, gasped, then vainly attempted to suppress her simultaneous shock and guffaw. For reasons best known only to herself, and possibly some of the fairies that occasionally flitted around her mind, Lady C. had decided that the appropriate course of action to prepare for this particular session of treatment, was to lie back on the traction bed, legs akimbo and stark naked, wearing nothing but her scarf (because she 'didn't want her neck to get chilly')!

From behind the (thankfully, visually-protective) curtain, all I could hear was Lady C. proffering, "I'm sorry my dear, I was only trying to help, I thought it might speed things up a bit, because I know how busy you all are."

That, along with the unmistakable sound of Jane, now attempting to stop the copious amounts of snot that were obviously firing out of her nostrils, as she valiantly, but vainly, attempted to suppress her laughter and maintain some vestige of decorum. Suitably re-dressed, Lady C. re-alighted onto the bed, Janet headed off to clean her face and life carried on as normal(ly as it could in that place).

CHAPTER 23

Professionally poor

Good reception and administrative staff are a godsend. A good team of front desk and back office workers is nigh-on worth its weight in gold, and I've had the good fortune to work with some of the best, absolute diamonds.

Unfortunately, I've also worked in a number of NHS hospital physiotherapy departments where admin' staff 'rule the roost', in some cases to the degree that they are, in effect and to all intents and purposes, clinically controlling the department. To be fair, it's sometimes been a case of 'needs must', in that the clinical staff present are for whatever reason(s) unable or unwilling to make the decisions needed to arrange and co-ordinate day-to-day patient lists.

I once worked in a South of England department where, due to the weakness and ineptitude of the Superintendent Physio' and Team Lead, the medically untrained administrative staff were, largely, unwillingly, forced into triaging and prioritising patient referrals and dictating appointment allocations.

As far as I am aware, from anecdotal, colleague-provided information, there is at least one such department where the practice continues still, to this day. Were the Care and Quality Commission (CQC) to visit, their inspectors would figuratively, if not quite literally, 'drop a bollock'! I witnessed an instance at this particular establishment which, colourfully and concisely, corroborated the above view, when a particularly unpleasant member of the reception team got her much-deserved come-uppance.

A patient had presented at the reception desk, to enquire as to why her young, teenage son had not yet received an appointment for treatment, despite him having been referred to the department for a physiotherapy consultation, some two months previously.

"We didn't feel he was a priority, as he's a young, healthy man and only had a minor injury," spat the condescending, patronising and big-mouthed receptionist, very cockily.

"Oh, I see," replied the mother, quietly and politely, "could you tell me who decided that please?"

"Well, I'm not sure, it could have been one of us, or one of the physiotherapists, depending on how complicated the referral seemed," said 'Cocky', setting herself up for the impending huge bear-trap, into which she was about to stomp.

"Oh, I see, And how, exactly, would you know of or ascertain its 'complexity'?!", asked the mother pointedly, and in a way that strongly suggested she might be somewhat medically informed.

"Er...well...er," faltered Cocky.

"Exactly!!!", snapped the mother abruptly, and with some considerable force, and then continued, "As you're so medically well informed, could you please tell me what's more serious, a fracture or a sprain?"

Now, at this point, if she'd possessed even a modicum of common sense, intuition or self-preservation, Cocky would've stopped digging that gargantuan hole she was already in, made her excuses and disappeared, to fetch someone who actually knew what they were talking about to deal with the situation. However, as well as being cocky, Cocky also had absolutely no ability to 'read the room', so, in true Darwinian, self-destructive, 'natural selection' style, she simply proceeded, assuredly and confidently, to answer thus.

"A fracture, obviously!"

"I see!" growled the mother, her eyes now narrowing like daggers, readying to skewer her hapless victim. And skewer she did. "So, a hairline fracture of a 5th metacarpal (wrist bone), on a non-dominant hand of a sedentary office worker would be more serious than a Grade 2 (moderate-serious) sprain of an anterior talo-fibular ligament (ATFL - big, strong ligament on the outside of the ankle), on a full-time working scaffolder, would it?!?!"

At this point even Cocky, dumb as she was, realised that she had massively bitten off far more than she could chew, was seriously out of her depth, and promptly went the colour of a beetroot in a jar of strawberry jam. She then rapidly scuttled off to find someone who might be able to equally, both answer and placate the now (justifiably) extremely irate mother.

It transpired that Mum was actually an Army Paramedic, who'd just returned from a tour of duty and, to be very frank, Cocky along with the head physiotherapist and hospital itself were all extremely lucky that she didn't lodge the, potentially very damaging, formal complaint which, at this point, she was seriously contemplating: Their collective arses would've been well and truly in a sling, and at least one P45 would quite likely have been thrown into the mix. As long as these sorts of situations are allowed to continue, there will almost certainly come a day when some poor soul of a patient, ends up seriously medically compromised, or indeed dead, due to the unqualified oversight, by an inept 'Cocky', of some critically important factor in their condition and/or treatment.

CHAPTER 24

CPD merry-go-round

Leading me, somewhat counter-intuitively, to expound on the vagaries (and also virtues, but mainly vagaries) of Continual Professional Development (CPD). A relatively important part of many professions, but one which in many has now grown exponentially to become, well, to put it bluntly, a self- perpetuating, money-making monster, that has seemingly lost sight of its original tenet.

It is now akin to a one-eyed gigantor, with its vision firmly fixed on the sole goal of wealth accumulation, and with many involved, making a very good living from the profits (some exceedingly so). This includes certain members of governing bodies/organisations' hierarchies, who are individually connected or associated in some way with said CPD Providers, in much the same way that many MPs varyingly profit, from associations with companies operating inside the very industries, or sectors, over which those very same MPs preside and legislate upon. It's a funny old World...

When vocational and professional practices alter, and techniques change substantially, within a particular discipline, then it is appropriate that the professional clinical workers involved are re-trained and re-educated appropriately, in order that they can up-skill themselves. So as to be able to avail their patients, or clients, of said (hopefully) superior and/or more efficacious treatment or service. However, if that 'new' technique, or clinical approach, is simply the 'rudimentary tweaking' or re-hashing of an already well established treatment method, or a moderately different view on a standard approach to an assessment/diagnostic protocol, then, in my view, it should not be made a mandatory skill, for which, poorly paid physiotherapists, have to shell-out a fair proportion of their hard earned income to (almost invariably) Third Party, corporate business-enterprises, in order to learn.

I'm a 'spinal specialist' physiotherapist, with 28 years' unbroken working experience, focusing on and treating spinal patients, occasionally resolving problems and issues that others (including APPs) have been unable to. I, along with a great number of my colleagues, am now towards 'the upper part of the tree' as regards clinical diagnosis, reasoning and treating abilities. Yet, despite this we, 'on paper', are considered to be professionally less-qualified, skilled or competent than those who have undertaken such aforementioned CPD courses, regardless of their 'true' levels of expertise. I include in the latter category those such as the previously mentioned inept Band 7 Senior Spinal Specialist Physiotherapist, or the Band 8 Team Lead Physiotherapist, who, despite all their (plentiful) certificates, and high-level title, was unable to comprehend that a 3cm discrepancy in a patient's leg length (right longer than left), could ultimately be the cause of their right arm pain (as a result of the bio-mechanical 'knock-on' effect, up their spine, causing additional postural problems 'higher up' and resulting in increased cervical [neck] nerve-root pressure with associated pain).

Regardless of one's religious, spiritual or evolutionary views, what most will likely admit is that the human body hasn't substantially changed in a very long time, thousands of years at least, and neither have its various tissue healing rates. Almost any physiotherapist with a sound grounding in and grasp of these tenets, along with that of a basic understanding of anatomy, physiology and biomechanics, together with cognisance of potential treatment dangers and/or contraindications, is likely going to remain efficient, effective, productive and safe throughout their career. A situation which can be easily and safely maintained with only minimal further formal training other than that gained via the (previously acknowledged to be) extremely effective method of direct work experience and tuition by senior colleagues.

CHAPTER 25

Symptom not the cause

Physiotherapists, general practitioners and consultants, myself included, are sometimes guilty of overlooking the obvious. If a patient says their pain in their shoulder 'feels like a toothache, i.e. a nerve-generated pain - pain caused by irritation of the nerve itself, as opposed to pain caused by irritation or damage to a muscle, bone or body part which that particular nerve connects to - then there's a really good chance it is just that, nerve/neural pain.

If pain doesn't resolve with localised, topical/symptomatic treatment, especially over a prolonged period, then there's a good chance that the source of the problem isn't actually in the area where the pain is being felt, but somewhere else. Such as at or near the spine, likely around the level of the spine which that particular nerve connects to. It's not rocket science, it's really not. Yet some practitioners, still, seem unable to 'connect the dots', or consider investigating such possibilities. The causes are often quite subtle, but equally, often, so are the solutions. Unfortunately, they can also, be slow to resolve, often too much so for many (practitioners and public alike).

A chronically (i.e. occurred over a long period) compressed nerve, isn't going to just 'pop back up' to its former state and recommence working it was before (the injury) the moment it's released. It'll more likely be similar to very slow-acting memory foam, re-forming back over days, weeks and sometimes months.

By the same token, nerves that are being subtly irritated, or compromised, don't always give instantaneous indications of such, quite rarely in fact. Yet, even today, some physiotherapists are still being taught to 'clear the neck/lower back' with quick checks, using quick, active movements. Meaning, that if the patient's shoulder, arm or leg pain and/or other symptoms cannot be immediately replicated with such movements, then, supposedly, 'a spinal issue cannot be the cause of the problem'.

I have never heard so much unmitigated rubbish in my life (except possibly during the occasional Parliamentary debate).

One of the better analogies I can give is, that if it rains heavily on Yr Wyddfa (Mount Snowdon) on a Saturday, it may not flood in Llanberis until the following Tuesday, but, 'sure as eggs are eggs', it's the same water that hit the mountain which is now causing the people to do their shopping in wellington boots!

Suddenly-experienced bodily pain, that is actually resultant from such minor, gradual-onset, nerve irritation, can be compared and paralleled with those bizarre and unpleasant office situations where, for no apparent reason, a worker suddenly jumps up and uncharacteristically shouts, punches, assaults or even kills their fellow worker(s), for no apparent reason. But it subsequently transpires that for months, years or even decades, they had been quietly, subtly and continually irritated, by some small stimuli/occurrence(s), the cumulative effect of which eventually results in triggering the event/pain.

Many injuries, symptoms and syndromes, from 'rotator cuff' (shoulder) pain, through 'carpal tunnel syndrome' (wrist pain) to 'chronic regional pain syndrome' (CRPS - pain over distinctly-bordered regions of the body) are attributable to this 'slow-burn', subliminal nerve(-root) irritation. Yet, again, I've seen patients undergo weeks, months, sometimes even years' worth of localised/symptomatic treatments - including massages, mobilisations, cortisone injections and surgeries - on these painful, isolated/localised body parts, all to no avail. Even then some practitioners continue on in the same vein, undeterred.

Sometimes in life the clues are so obvious that they're hiding in plain sight, and possibly that's why they are so often missed. As one, seasoned CIA operative, purportedly once said, "Never in history has there been such a deadly missed clue as when the '911' Al-Qaeda terrorist pilot, whilst being trained to fly, stated to his military-trained instructor that he 'didn't need to learn how to land'!"

With regard to the above, on a very precise lumbar spinal (lower back) note, and as a general 'heads-up' – which, if it aids even just one physio' to in turn help just one patient resolve their pain, will have been worth mentioning - when it comes to referred-pain and symptoms, physiotherapists (and doctors) sometimes fail to take into account the importance of the lumbar spine, L2 (upper part) level, specifically the L2 Dorsal Root Lateral Ganglions. A seemingly innocuous pair of little nerve bundles, tucked away on either side of the L2 vertebra). These two little nerve lumps are super-sensitive and, even from only the slightest of irritations (e.g. pressure from poor lumbar-posture), can be extremely reactive, causing disproportionately large amounts of localised and/or referred pain and symptoms, into the buttocks, hips and lower limbs. The number of instances of undiagnosed pain and symptoms that these two little organs are likely responsible for is impossible to calculate. But if you happen to have a patient with an as-yet undiagnosed aetiology (origin) of such pain(s), and for whom other treatments haven't worked, then gently mobilising their upper lumbar spine and correcting their lumbar posture might well be very beneficial. I've truly lost count of the number of athletes and sportspeople who, over the years, have had numerous, frequent calf and hamstring tears or, sadly, career-ending complete ruptures, when their injury-causing problem has actually been elsewhere in their body. The injury having simply been a distal (distant) symptom, of a central (spinal) problem.

There remain to this day many, including some top athletes, whose problem(s) could likely be rapidly resolved, and chances of re-injury possibly almost completely negated, by the most basic of assessments, simplest of treatments and easiest of exercises. A moderately bright guy, by the name of Albert Einstein, once said, "The definition of insanity, is doing the same thing over and over and expecting a different result". If he's right, then unfortunately there are a fair few of us who could well be candidates for membership of the 'coats that fasten-up at the back' club!

* * *

Technical case in point: Top rugby player who suffered repeatedly from right leg, hamstring strains and tears, together with frequent pain of varying levels in the back of his right thigh.

He sought treatment from all quarters, but to no avail, with the injuries gradually increasing in both frequency and severity, to the point where they were impacting upon the guy's chances of furthering his career and possibly gaining an international cap. Short version: I assessed the man, ascertained that the aetiology (origin) of his problem was a very heavy kick to the thigh, that he'd received some years earlier. I treated his right quadricep (specifically rectus femoris - big, front-thigh muscle) and resolved his problem.

Long version: The historic kick had caused severe contusion to the guy's right quad muscle (rectus femoris), which, in reaction, had proceeded to slowly but surely, markedly tighten and shorten. This tight muscle had then pulled on and torsioned his right-sided pelvic bone (ilium), in turn causing a tightness on the right- side of his lumbar spine, with subsequent right-sided nerve root irritation. That resulted in abnormal signals travelling down the right sciatic nerve, causing the right hamstrings to repeatedly tighten and contract incorrectly, culminating in the patient's hamstring problem/muscle injury. I know this to be the case, because I only treated and lengthened the man's right quad' muscle - with deep massage, acupressure and basic stretching techniques - and the man's chronic pain completely disappeared, within the space of 10 days.

'Lourdes'

With regard to the above, a very recent, quite apt, somewhat serious case in point. I assessed a patient in his early forties, who'd been referred to the physiotherapy department by a consultant neurologist, simply for the supply and fitting of an ankle splint, to correct his 'foot drop'. This problem had arisen due to 'permanent' physiological nerve damage/deterioration, of unknown origin, in this patient's leg. 'Foot drop' is a clinical condition, whereby the patient has a 'floppy' foot, due to damage to the (common peroneal) nerve controlling the calf/ankle muscles that pull up (dorsiflex) their ankles/feet/toes. Meaning that they are unable to actively lift their foot up or pull it back, making walking very difficult, as the whole leg has to be raised up much higher than normal, whilst stepping forwards, in order to ensure the foot clears the ground and doesn't catch, as it swings forward.

People with this condition tend to look like walking flamingos, with their high-stepping gait. This particular patient had already been allocated his splint - Ankle-Foot Orthosis (AFO) splint and also been told that this was how he would have to (learn to) walk for the rest of his life. It was a simple, 'prescriptive' type, 'splint-fitting and exercise-only' referral from the consultant, as he had deemed the patient's injury and status to be irreversible. However, true to form, despite the consultant's definitive diagnosis and prognosis, I decided to perform my normal New Patient Assessment on the man.

After close examination, I felt that things simply 'didn't add up', especially regarding the patient's history of symptom onset (HPC), especially given the fact that they had experienced prolonged periods of varying-level low back pain, at around the time their 'foot-drop' symptom(s) had commenced. I subsequently concluded that the patient's nerve had simply been contused and compressed, at its root, in the foraminal area (entry to the spine).

Long story short; after 3 weeks of lumbar spine treatment and specific, proprioceptive neuromuscular facilitation (PNF) exercises, the patient went from 0/5 ('no movement/strength') to 5/5 ('full movement/strength'), i.e. complete recovery, with normal foot/ankle movements and full walking ability.

The neurosurgeon involved was dutifully informed of the findings, treatment and conclusion, but no response was forthcoming.

The most worrying and somewhat ominous aspect of this case is, that if the patient had used the splint, his relevant dorsiflexion muscles would have suffered 'disuse atrophy' and eventually 'dissolved away'. This, perversely, would eventually have actually resulted in the patient becoming 'genuinely' permanently disabled, in a quite unedifying variation of a 'self-fulfilling prophecy'.

CHAPTER 26

Plain nasty

The majority of physiotherapists are pleasant, affable, helpful people, often willing to go 'the extra mile' to help patients and colleagues alike. Unfortunately, there is a small group of physiotherapists, all of a certain ilk, who are the complete antitheses of this. They're predominantly, almost exclusively, female, of a certain age, middle-class, generally hail from the Home Counties and seem to harbour resentment towards, well, just about everybody, but especially anyone they perceive to be 'doing better than them', at pretty much anything at all really.

It's a very destructive type of unpleasantness and quite a 'sight to behold', when unleashed in any of its many guises. I've been the target of a few such attacks over the course of my career, but have thankfully, generally been able to repel and quickly neutralise them on almost every occasion. Mainly because the assaults are almost invariably passive-aggressive in nature, and therefore tend to 'stop dead' at 'neutral brick wall' or 'active combative' responses. I've always thought passive-aggression to be 'go to' of cowards, the insecure and those of low moral fibre.

Sadly, I witnessed from afar, this particular form of unpleasantness being employed and deployed upon others, on (far too) many occasions. I've usually intervened when it seemed appropriate and where I've been able, but have always been cognisant of (and moderated by) the fact that, sometimes, by getting involved, I could be making things worse in the long-term, for the targeted individual.

I clearly remember one such situation in a Physiotherapy Department at a large hospital in SW England. Caroline was a nice, very nice - probably her biggest 'fault', as most of the 'passive-aggressive, chipped-shoulder brigade' tend to especially dislike very nice people, probably because such niceness highlights their own true, unpleasant natures - physio', in her late 50s.

On this particular day she was in a bit of a bind, because, through no fault of her own, she'd over-run on her morning, inpatient clinical duties and was now very severely pushed for time, with her afternoon outpatient treatment list. It was clearly apparent to all the other physiotherapists in the office (three plus myself), that this long-term, permanent member of their own team was extremely stressed, yet none of them even enquired as to what the (very obvious) problem was, never mind offered to help. Furthermore, it was obvious to me that, at least two of them were actually deriving pleasure from Caroline's predicament, in a very 'schaudenfreudy' sort of way. This included one particular grouch, who had at least two hours treatment-time free, having been fortuitous enough to have just had three, concurrent patients from her afternoon treatment list, cancel their appointments in quick succession (I'm pretty-sure they did so in the hope of being re-booked with a different physio', for this person was truly, a thoroughly unpleasant individual).

I went over to Caroline, told her I had one empty slot, with one likely 'quick check-up' type of patient immediately afterwards, and asked if I could help, by taking on one of her current patients.

"No, it's ok, I think I'll be alright, but thank you," she said, quietly, and then, as I turned to walk away, Caroline caught my arm, looked me in the eye and with what I can only describe as a combined expression of pain, upset and resignation whispered, "You know, I've worked here almost 10 years and no one's ever offered to help me like that."

It was, professionally one of the saddest things I'd ever heard. Things shouldn't be like that in the World generally and certainly not in one of a 'caring' profession like Physiotherapy. Unfortunately however 'there's how it should be and there's how it is'. How and why people become so unpleasant is obviously a combination of nature, nurture and experience, though I do believe that some people are simply 'born nasty'.

CHAPTER 27

Tesco commandos

Now I don't know what it is about physiotherapists and our profession, but we seem to be unique in the fact that, unlike any other allied health or medical profession in the World, our patients seem to have no inhibitions (and indeed feel it a natural right or duty) in regaling us with 'situation-reports' on the recovery-stage or otherwise of their respective ailments, whenever they happen to meet us outside of the clinical setting, regardless of the setting or circumstance. Nowhere, it seems, is off limits.

I once had a patient quiz me at length on the likely progress of his injury-recovery, as we progressed (far too slowly) towards the sales cashier in a cinema queue - thankfully he was waiting to see a different film to myself and partner, otherwise I swear he'd have continued questioning me right up to the start of the film, if not actually during it!

Another episode occurred whilst I was sitting having a quiet, romantic coffee with my girlfriend, at a park cafe one

Sunday morning. On spotting me, the man in question actually made a massive swerve, detour and back-track from his intended walking route, in order to interrupt and subsequently foist upon us, a debrief of his current injury status and rehab' exercise schedule.

"That shooting pain, down the left side of my back and into my buttock has eased-off, and the groin pain's gone completely, so the exercises are obviously helping, but I wondered if I could just quickly ask you...?!"

You never hear of people approaching their local GP in WH Smiths and saying, "Oh doctor, that haemorrhoid cream you gave me doesn't seem to be working at the moment", or enquiring of their Gynaecologist, on the Tube, whether or not their smear test results are ready. Yet many feel it's fine to importune upon their physio', any time or place.

It's this sort of predicament that resulted in Kev and myself instigating our once-weekly 'commando raids' on the local Tesco-Extra supermarket. The objective was, to make it into the store, do our weekly shopping and get out again without being accosted by any patient(s), in any way, shape or form. Given that the supermarket in question was the closest, indeed only (proper), one in our hospital's very large catchment area, this was no easy task. So difficult in fact, that in a 6-month period we didn't manage it even once, regardless of the time we chose to shop.

One particular Saturday morning, Kev and I had got to the shop very, very early and, having made it all the way round without bumping into a single patient (despite the shop still being remarkably busy for that time of day), were now highly confident of at last 'breaking our duck' and making it out unassailed.

As our goods moved down adjacent checkout belts and neared the cashier point, ready to be processed, we turned to look at each other, gave mutual, childish 'double thumbs-ups' and laughed. We'd made it!

At that precise moment my laugh stopped, my jaw and eyes opened in mock shock, and my head turned, with an almost imperceptible, simultaneous nod, indicating to Kev that she should look behind her. Kev began to comedically turn her whole body, head frozen in position, eyes starting to widen in true sit-com style, as the hand from behind simultaneously landed on her shoulder.

"Oh 'ello, fancy seeing you 'ere," said one of Kev's patients, "glad I did though. Y'know I've done everything you said, but my shoulder's still quite painful...!"

Tesco's had defeated us once again!!!

CHAPTER 28

Critical incident

Within the medical world a 'Critical Incident' is one which requires notification of its event to the appropriate, concerned governing body. Almost every health worker will encounter and experience at least one in their career, and they range from the minor to the major, and from relatively routine to completely bizarre, the latter definitely being the applicable category in the following case. I'd just attempted to open the front door of the Physiotherapy department on a Monday morning and found it was already unlocked.

"Oh, Geoff the (hydrotherapy) pool-man must already be here," I said to Rebecca, as we walked through the wide bay door which opened straight into the gymnasium area.

"Maybe he is, but I don't think that should be!", said Rebecca, having stopped dead in her tracks, now pointing pointedly and wide-eyed, at the massive, quite literally 'donkey-sized' black dildo, standing proudly erect on the first-bay treatment bed!

“Wow! Did you not take all your stuff home on Friday?!?!”, I said jokingly, in surprise and bewildered bemusement.

Fifteen seconds later, after surviving an intense, but thankfully short-lived admonishing stare-attack from Rebecca, that would honestly have made Godzilla fill his pants, we both continued, now somewhat trepidatiously, towards the office and entrance of the hydrotherapy pool.

“Just hang on here a sec’ Bec,” I said, nodding towards the pool door, having concluded on quick inspection that the glass-doored, small office was empty, and also noting the half-empty bottle of baby oil on the floor, next to the entrance. “HELLOOOOO! IF ANYONE’S IN THERE I SUGGEST YOU FUCK OFF THROUGH THE EMERGENCY DOOR, RIGHT NOW,!!!THE COPS ARE ON THEIR WAY AND I’VE GOT AN IRON BAR!!!” (I actually did have, though it was more of a bendy pole really; the one we used to close the top louvre windows in the gym).

I entered the hydro pool area, slowly and cautiously, but thankfully the room was empty. “Rebecca, you’d better get in here!”, I shouted. She did so, and our collective mood instantly plummeted, from somewhat excitable bemusement to extreme concern. Scattered around the pool were various pieces of clothing, some lingerie, a riding crop, a couple of used condoms, a ‘film script/prompter’..... and a pile of children’s clothing!

“Oh god I feel sick!”, whispered Becs.

“I’ll call the police. Don’t touch anything and walk the exact line out that you walked in!”, I said, now in a very different head-space to the one I’d left home in, only 20 minutes earlier.

Though located within a city, this particular clinic was a remote satellite, of the main hospital that Rebecca and I worked for. Locationally relatively isolated and, being unoccupied on weekends, somewhat susceptible to such potential illegal-entry type incidents. What occurred next was like something out of the opening scene of a 1980s action movie!

The police arrived first, screeching into the car park, skidding to a halt and exiting their cars with a speed and gusto normally reserved for entering the local doughnut shop. I was actually a bit disappointed that at least one of them didn’t commando-roll into a bush and shout, “Freeze!”

Next came the ambulance, obviously being driven by someone thinking they were about to be the first responder at a Jumbo Jet crash site, given the side-lean he produced in the van as he turned to enter the gates. He was closely followed by, equally, one of the fastest fire engines I’ve ever seen, and certainly the only one ever to have (momentarily) ridden on two wheels, as it too swooped in through the entrance and then cranked the turn even harder, in order to avoid the now stationary ambulance - its presence due to the fact that, as I was speaking to the emergency switchboard operator on the phone, Rebecca, obviously within earshot, had piped up, "I think I can smell gas too". Having forgotten that we often could, sporadically, as a result of the gym's antiquated air-conditioning unit, but it wasn't the combustible sort. The operator had, quite correctly, obviously unilaterally acted upon this info'.

Next came the bods from social services, all 'yoghurts, Crocs and hemp trousers', in their hospital-issue people-carrier, looking like they were actually trying their level-best to live up to some sort of 70s comedic stereotype.

Then came the detectives, from the Special Investigations Unit and Vice Squad. A subsequent, continual conga-line of Health Authority officials followed thereafter, each incrementally more senior than the one before them, until the head honcho, the big boss herself turned up. She was a short, squat, somewhat gruff woman, whom I'd heard of, but never met before, and eerily reminiscent of former British MP, Anne Widdecombe, not only in stature, but outlook and demeanour too. She was reputedly a bit of a 'tough cookie', administratively at least, but that reputation went south faster than a stripper's knickers the moment she stepped into the gym!

'Anne' took one look at the 'donkey-dildo', squeaked like a demented mouse, spun around and headed straight back out the door, as fast as her little, jelly-like legs could carry her - gibbering and muttering as she fled. One of the nearby, female police detectives nearly choked, and simultaneously coughed and farted, in her efforts to suppress the uncontrollable laughter that had instantly enveloped her body (I remember it as if it were yesterday). Normally ultra-reserved Rebecca, shot off in the opposite direction, straight back into the crime scene and towards the office, at warp speed, doubled-over, hand on mouth, visibly convulsing with mirth. I simply stood and tactfully laughed out loud, doing nothing to try and disguise my amusement, other than turn slightly away from the rapidly moving moon-bear - quite possibly why I never received any promotions from that day forth.

A few patients whom we hadn't been able to contact in time arrived and quickly left again, with instructions to call the next day for further appointments. Rebecca and I were repeatedly questioned by various officials and officers, had our fingerprints taken as exculpatory evidence and, around early afternoon, were given the rest of the day off.

Because of the children's clothing and 'minors' aspect to the case, and everything that it potentially implied, the investigation was given top priority. The police threw everything but the kitchen sink at it.

It transpired that our clinic had been used to make several hardcore pornography films, with a 'doctor & nurse themes', over that weekend, all of which were actually completed and distributed within three days of the incident, but were equally quickly, sourced, located and confiscated by the police.

The silver lining to the cloud, was that the clothing hadn't been intended for children at all, but in fact been used by very small, diminutive young women from South-East Asia, all of whom had starring roles in the various film storylines.

We think Moon-bear Anne subsequently had to have a fair bit of counselling, for PTSD. By all accounts she was definitely not 'herself' for a good few weeks!

You often get them in physio', the 'I bet you didn't think your day was going to turn out like this when you got out of bed this morning' type scenarios, but this day definitely ranked right up there, near the very top of the list.

CHAPTER 29

It's a locum thing

I've worked as a permanent physiotherapist, in long-term NHS/Public Health posts and as a locum physio', both here in the UK and abroad, and have found that attitudes towards locum staff (in the UK specifically) range right across the spectrum of sentiments. From those who embrace the locum(s) and are grateful for their services (even to the degree of some allowing locums to join in with their in-service training courses), through to those who, quite literally, seem to despise them, viewing their presence as a 'necessary evil', to be begrudgingly tolerated.

Certain politicians seem to fall into this latter category and I personally have no truck with them or their sentiments, finding them moronically myopic in their outlook. What they seem to forget is that without locum staff the National Health Service would likely almost collapse. I personally have lost count of the number of times when, working as a locum, I've been accused of 'having it better than the permanent staff', with 'much more pay, less responsibility and a generally easier work-life'. My replies to such neg-heads have always remained steadfastly the same: The long version goes, "If you take into account the paid holidays, paid sick leave, paid extra bank holidays and paid parental leave that you receive and which I, as a locum worker, don't, then factor in the travel and weekly accommodation costs that I have to pay and you don't, I think you'll find that you're actually 'streets ahead' of me financially. Plus, every locum position is by nature temporary, insecure, socially isolating and instantly terminable at any time, with only one day's notice, so all in all not the 'great gig' it's made out to be.

The short version goes; "If it's such a great a job why don't you stop whinging and do it yourself?!"

My first ever job as a locum was at a hospital where staffing levels were so low, due to terrible staff retention and attrition rates as a result of appalling management, that on two separate occasions, we seven locums (of nine total staff) had to sit in a circle and pass our weekly time-sheets 'one to the right', to counter-sign each other's 'confirmation of hours worked'. This situation was not the 'fault' of the locums, nor of the staff, but that of the departmental and hospital management as a whole'.

Locums, by the very nature of their job remit, usually get to see a broad spectrum of hospitals, clinics, health facilities and associated work venues, from the very best to the very worst, and are therefore uniquely placed to potentially advise on how things could, or should, be changed for the better. It's something that some politicians might want to consider and possibly embrace, rather continuously beat down on them like some sort of demented Flintstones 'Bam-Bam'.

CHAPTER 30

Don't mess with your physio'

Kev was kicking back in her office during a break, feet up on her radiator, cuppa in hand, chatting on the phone. All was well with the world…..until the girl entered her office; a stumbling, mumbling, teary-eyed ball of upset!

"What's up, what's happened?!", exclaimed Kev, extremely concerned at the visible girl's state.

The young physio' paused, blurted out the sequence of events that had led to her current state of upset and despair, then immediately proceeded to recommence her sobbing.

"Gotta go Mum, speak soon, love yuh!", said Kev, rapidly hanging up the phone and then, turning to the still sobbing girl, placed a hand gently on the youngster's shaking shoulder, guided her towards the door and said quietly, "C'mon chicken, we've got a muppet to sort out."

On entering the ward Kev could see her adversary (for that is indeed, unfortunately, what he was) standing at the foot of the patient's bed, surrounded by a group of subservient 'underlings' - nurses, junior doctors, junior registrars, senior registrars; a veritable old-school 'ward-round flotilla' - together with another physiotherapist, who was currently the latest target receiving a full-frontal assault of admonishment from said adversary, the consultant orthopaedic surgeon, Mr 'Gobshite'.

Kev quickened her pace, walked up to the tall, angry man, drew herself up to her full 5'2" height and asked politely, "What seems to be the problem Mr G.?"

"Problem!!?!!", exploded the consultant, "Problem?! I'll tell you what the problem is!!!" he thundered.

"Ooh yes, please do, yuh cockwomble!", thought Kev, eyes fixed intently on the fuming red-faced man.

"Your damn staff are NOT doing their job, THAT'S the problem!!! I want THAT man (pointing to the 140kg+/22 stone patient, lying in the reinforced bariatric bed) out of his bed and into that chair, NOW!!! He needs to be mobilised after his total hip replacement and it's YOUR physio's' job to do it!"

"Yes, you're right," replied Kev quietly, "but there's the health and safety aspect to consider here. That gentleman's extremely heavy and there's no way that my two members of staff can safely help him transfer out from his bed to his chair on their own. And as there are no other qualified bodies available to assist, we've got a bit of a problem!"

"THEN GET MORE STAFF!", said the cockwomble, at the top of his voice. Then, drawing himself up to his full height, he shouted, "I don't care how many of you it takes I..... WANT....THAT.... MAN....OUT…OF…BED…NOW!!!"

Gobshite was a very prickly, tricky character, with somewhat of a reputation throughout the hospital for being, well, there's no other way to put it, an uncooperative, arrogant arsehole of the first order, who was relentless in getting things his own way and 'didn't take prisoners', so Kev had to tread a little carefully. Unfortunately for the cockwomble, Kev had missed the 'diplomatic brown-nosing of consultants' section in her induction package, when she started working at that particular hospital.

"Now, right now?", repeated Kev, through gritted teeth, eyes fixed on Mr G. like a mongoose sizing up a snake. "Hmmm, ok, leave it with me, I'll be back in a minute." And with that Kev strode off, making sure to drag her two charges along with her and well out of cockwomble's fire-zone.

Fifteen minutes later Gobshite's jaw (and everyone else's for that matter) hit the floor with a veritable thud, as four, fully kitted-out firemen, preceded by Kev, walked onto the ward and up to the moribund patient's bed. Expertly supervised by Kev, the three men and one woman from Trumpton deftly, swiftly and gently helped the man transfer out of his bed and into his chair, with a couple of interim small, assisted, weight-bearing exercise-steps and mini-squats mid-move, for good measure. The firemen all wished the patient well, smiled, turned to face

Kev, saluted her in unison and left. Kev turned to the cock-womble, who still bore an expression like he'd just seen the cat ordering a takeaway pizza, pointed her finger at him and said, through still gritted teeth and in a tone that would have scared Hannibal Lecter, "Now YOU can get him back in to his bed when the time comes, because my staff aren't going to. And don't you EVER bully any of my staff, EVER again, EVER!!!"

Kev marched off, ...and he never did, ever!

To this day no one knows 'who or how', but that day Kev became an official legend.

CHAPTER 31

Don't shoot the messenger

Amongst other things, physiotherapists are one of the professions most at risk of suffering the effects from 'Pheidippides Syndrome' (PS) - according to Greek legend Pheidippides was the first person to run the marathon distance, from the town of Marathon to Athens, delivering a war victory message - or more accurately 'Shooting the Messenger Syndrome' (SMS).

PS/SMS occur frequently in medical settings but especially so in physiotherapy, because our work often involves us having to deliver news that people really don't want to hear and, in response, for reasons best known to themselves, those same people often 'let rip' at us, the physiotherapists.

It's not that we're even trying to 'play devil's advocate' (an expression and position that I personally am often a bit suspicious of), but simply giving people very basic, factual information about their condition, situation or problem, and the best, sometimes the only, way for them to go about resolving it. Much of which, frequently, they already, honestly know to be the case, but possibly simply don't want to have to acknowledge or contemplate it.

CHAPTER 32

Practice what you preach

As physiotherapists we have to interact with doctors on an almost daily basis and, as with physiotherapists, they come in all varieties of personality, attitude and competence. Unfortunately however, many doctors have gone the way of the general population, in managing to pile on the pounds, despite their having far better knowledge than most as regards the bad health effects of doing so. So widespread now is this obesity problem within the medical profession, that an emergency 'crash call' can sometimes resemble something like Colonel Heffa's, Jungle Book Patrol, clattering down corridors, bumping along, as they trundle rather than run to the stricken patient(s).

Back in the 1980s and 90s, I knew of at least three junior house officers (junior/resident doctors) who were owed numerous debts of gratitude, by people that they had been able to successfully resuscitate and bring back to life, purely as a result of said doctors' abilities to run the 400m length of that particular hospital in less than 90 seconds, …whilst carrying a heavy resuscitation-bag and negotiating 25-30 stairs in the process.

Physiotherapists, generally, have not yet succumbed to the creeping advance of widespread weight gain, and still tend to lead by example, especially in outpatient departments - it's pretty hard to convincingly preach the 'fit and healthy' mantra to someone, if you're far less fit than they, or indeed a wobbling dough ball.

I once witnessed such an event in the physiotherapy gymnasium of a West London hospital. The very large physiotherapist was trying to demonstrate some knee, muscle-strengthening and proprioceptive-control exercises, to a very fit-looking and quite motivated patient. As big-boy explained what needed to be done, the patient stared at him with expressions that ranged from incredulity to complete blankness, and understandably so, given that, due to his size and lack of fitness, the physiotherapist in question was actually unable to accurately demonstrate or, in one, case even perform the exercises. Even whilst obviously still quite significantly injured, this patient was able to outperform the physiotherapist in each and every exercise.

Opinions are like arseholes, almost everyone has one, a few are quite shitty and some really stink, but for what it's worth, mine is simply this, that as far as health, fitness and exercise rehab' are concerned, wherever possible, physiotherapists need to lead by example.

CHAPTER 33

Coincidently Jamaican rumbled

There is a saying, well, combined 'utterance and action' really, that emanates from Jamaica and the rest of the West Indies, which is the 'ultimate in contempt'. It's called 'kissing your teeth' and is the Caribbean equivalent of calling someone a 'See you next Tuesday' in English. It really is that offensive.

The full action of 'kissing your teeth', involves the act of very audibly inhaling and sucking air into one's mouth, through clenched teeth, with lips pushed against them, restricting the air-flow, causing the distinctive sound, whilst simultaneously uttering the words 'raas klaart'. In Jamaican dialect, 'raas' means 'a woman's vagina', and 'klaart' means 'blood clot'. So calling someone a 'raas klaart', actually means you're saying they're equal to the clotted blood from a woman's menstrual cycle. Like many insults, the epithet often gets shortened. In this case, it's reduced down to just a short, but loud 'teeth kiss'; unmistakable in sound and losing none of its meaning or inference. In (specifically) Jamaican and 'West Indian' culture, it is probably the ultimate (misogynistic) insult, though it's also sometimes used as a very strong indication, of extreme annoyance at, or dislike of, a particular person, comment or action.

I once saw a Jamaican woman slap a man, so hard that he fell over, simply (and rightly) because he had inadvertently (but instinctively, as a reflex reaction) 'kissed his teeth' at her, in reaction to a verbal slight from said woman. The man subsequently stood back up, and did precisely nothing. He knew he'd 'crossed-the-line' and gotten his (extremely) just deserts.

I know (very reliably) second hand, of a young, 12-year-old boy, who received a 'backhander' to the face from his mother, hard enough to knock him sideways off his chair and onto the ground, numerous times in quick succession, on the basis of performing said insult.

So comfortable was the boy with using said expression, that he had done so inadvertently, as an unconscious, reflex reaction, to what he perceived as a verbal sleight from one of his teachers. Who, at the time, was admonishing the boy in front of his mother at a pre-arranged 'intervention', necessitated by the boy's ever-declining standard of behaviour at school.

At home he was, seemingly, an 'absolute angel', 'mummy's little cherub' in fact. At school, it was a very different matter, with him 'kissing his teeth' at will, towards anyone and everyone who vexed or irritated him in any way whatsoever. Some would say 'abuse', 'shouldn't have happened', 'wrong'; others, the opposite. I say, there's the idealistic, 'how it should be', and there's the realistic, how it is.

How it should be: he was spoken to, sternly and with gravitas, in order to educate and make him fully aware as to the error of his ways. Repeatedly so and at length, enough that he changed his behaviour and stopped doing it.

How it is: the lad experienced a short, sharp and harsh, but very valuable lesson (and what transpired to be a 'watershed moment' in his life) in what sort of behaviour is absolutely unacceptable (in a[lmost any] given situation).

It truly was a watershed moment for the boy. Prior to it, he had been on a life-pathway that was likely going to see him expelled from school and all that often subsequently entails. Subsequent to it, he buckled up his ideas, knuckled down, became a 'star pupil' and ended up going to university.

As regards 'wrong'. Well, for what it's worth, and possibly a little controversially, 'philosophically' speaking, there is no such thing as (absolute) right or wrong, only 'degrees of opinion, on any particular point, in any particular place, at any particular place in time'. If you doubt it, put it to the test, regarding anything. I once did so in discussion with a friend, on a (to him) very sensitive topic about a historical world event. He said that it shouldn't have happened (and I totally agree/d) and was totally wrong. I simply said that at that place/point, the (consensus of opinion) was that it was 'right', ...because it happened, intentionally! Mind you, 'Schrodinger's cat style', that's only my opinion.

These days though, like so many others, the insult is so prolifically overused that its impact and derisory effect has been somewhat diluted, but it has to be said, in this particular case, not a lot. My reason for relaying this piece of (no doubt stultifying) information, is that it informs and enlightens upon the following short story.

The highly experienced and specialised physiotherapist was called Natasha, and so skilled was she in her particular field, that her help with patients was frequently called upon, from far and wide, by many of her colleagues and fellow professionals. Only a few days prior to the following occurrence I had, coincidentally, been explaining all about 'kissing the teeth' to Nats, in response to comments and questions she'd made about it, having seen and heard the insult being delivered by someone, during a television documentary programme, a few days earlier. Natasha had been totally nonplussed and somewhat shocked, by the insult recipient's violent reaction to the insult itself.

On this particular day, Natasha had been requested to fly off and treat someone at a very distant location to her hometown, another country in fact. It transpired that the elderly patient was originally from the Caribbean and, unbeknownst to

Natasha at the time, was also the mother of a quite, well, very, famous person. Natasha approached the well-presented and highly alert elderly woman, sitting up in her hospital bed.

"Hello Mrs X, I'm Natasha, 'Nats' to my friends, and I've been sent here to see if I can help you at all, if you're happy for me to do so of course?!", chirped Nats, pleasantly.

"Oh, ok, no problem," smiled Mrs X, "do what you have to do young lady."

"Great, will do," replied Nats. "First I'll have to ask you a few questions and then, once that's done, we can have a look and see what we can possibly do to help you."

Nats proceeded with her assessment of Mrs X and, all was going swimmingly, until it happened! Suddenly, as a result of a momentary shot of pain, inadvertently caused by Nats gently lifting the lady's arm, Mrs X recoiled and pulled her arm away, whilst simultaneously and instinctively kissing her teeth at Natasha! It was now Nats turn to 'recoil', in perfect, comedic, melodramatic style!!!

It has to be noted at this point, that Nats was a consummate comedian. Able to, gently but amusingly, make light of almost any situation and frequently leave all around her in stitches, with an amazing range of funny voices, expressions and body-morphs. "DID YOU JUST KISS YOUR TEETH AT ME?! DID YOU JUST KISS YOUR TEETH AT ME 'YOUNG' LADY?!" cried Nats, employing her best mock-shock voice and expression. "MY BEST FRIEND NATHAN TOLD ME ONLY LAST WEEK EXACTLY WHAT THAT MEANS! I THINK YOU'VE SOME EXPLAINING TO DO! I THINK YOU'RE GOING TO HAVE TO WORK VERY HARD TO REDEEM YOURSELF NOW!", she continued, in a fashion that had both attending nurses immediately in stitches, and Mrs X slightly unsure as to whether she should laugh or look suitably contrite.

"Ooh, Mum, been caught out this time, haven't you?! Didn't think a white person would know what you meant did you? I've told you about that before, and now you've been caught out, eh? Serves you right, Mum!" Mrs X's expression instantly turned to one of acute shame and embarrassment.

Natasha whipped her head round to see a very famous face (VFF) peering around the door, sporting a big, beaming smile. On having been informed about what had happened to their mother, 'VFF' had immediately jetted in to see her.

"Oh, gosh, I'm so sorry, I didn't know you were there!", said Nats, slightly contritely.

"Nooo, please don't apologise, it's high time someone pulled mum up on this. She occasionally does it, only to white people though, because she knows that they won't understand. I've already told her off about this sort of behaviour quite a few times in the past, but obviously she's never listened. I think she will now though, WON'T YOU MUM!?", said the

VFF, turning slightly to face their parent. Mrs X lowered her gaze, opened her eyes amusingly wide and, with just the hint of a guilty smile, gently nodded.

VFF then stayed for another half an hour or so, to chat with their mother, quiz Nats about various factors associated with their mum's likely treatment and recovery prognosis, thank the now somewhat awe-struck nurses and then left.

Mrs X went on to make a speedy and full recovery and, safe to say, did not kiss her teeth or indeed even inhale strongly, even once, for the rest of her stay.

CHAPTER 34

Be careful who you trust

I worked for a well-known UK Locum Agency for seven years, on one occasion saving them from a situation so serious (and similar to one already mentioned) that, if unresolved, it would almost certainly have led to said agency being seriously sanctioned and possibly resulted in loss of their NHS accreditation. Yet, during the recent pandemic, at the first sign of this agency having to incur the slightest temporary cost on my behalf, and despite my unbroken, diligent (and arse-saving) service, they dropped me like the proverbial stone - within 24 hours - causing me prolonged and severe financial hardship.

When the company CEO was subsequently informed of the situation (and reminded of the fact that, were it not for my actions he might not currently have a company), the best he could offer by way of thanks and reparations, was 'a meal out somewhere once things return to normal'.

Many medical staff supply companies (and other organisations in general) like this, often express annoyance and incredulity at the seeming fickleness and lack of loyalty displayed by many of their employees. Yet in many cases, it's simply a case of quid pro quo!

A timely addendum to the above. To any current physiotherapist(s) reading this, please note well, that you'd be very well advised to join a trade union - in addition to the Chartered Society of Physiotherapists (CSP) - a single-focus union, i.e. one whose sole remit and task is to protect and support you as an individual and independent practitioner.

Many physiotherapists seem to be unaware of the fact that, within the CSP there are two separate departments, both serviced by CSP employees and governed by the CSP hierarchy. One (rightly) oversees the upkeep of professional standards, and the other deals with the legal defence of any physio' unfortunate enough to be accused of (amongst other things) professional misconduct or breaching professional standards' rules. Thus, in any such given case, the former-cited office would be helping the Health Care Professions Council (HCPC - official governing body for professional standards across all allied health professions) in 'prosecuting' you, whilst the latter-cited department would be tasked with 'defending' you. This is, quite literally, the perfect description of a 'conflict of interests'!!!

I have had the misfortune to have witnessed second and third (but thankfully as yet not first) hand***** a number of legal tribunal cases. I can say is without fear of contradiction, that if there is choice, between protecting you as a practitioner (personally and professionally), or protecting/saving of the 'good name'/reputation of the organisation(s) involved, then, tragically, sister/ brother/other, you are almost certainly 'going under the bus'!

This is one of the few areas in which organisations are truly egalitarian, in that, regardless of race, colour, creed, class, religion or gender, if 'push comes to shove', they will seemingly happily 'sacrifice' any individual, ...and at a dizzying rate of knots.

*****Though in these days of seeming hyper-vigilance, extra-sensitivity and instant litigation - with the latter being many's 'instant default mode' - every health practitioner would seem to be only 'one step away' from such, regardless of their professional integrity, performance or conduct.

CHAPTER 35

Defy the odds

I was in a large, spacious and very brightly lit gym, with approximately 30 of the toughest, fittest, most focused and 'no nonsense' type individuals as you are ever likely to meet together in one room, at the same time. Men and women alike, including five of the biggest, meanest-looking and likely most hairy-arsed blokes on the planet.

We were dutifully awaiting arrival of the physiotherapist who, to cover for a sick colleague, had been assigned and transferred at the last moment to step in and lead this group, in a week-long session of 'injury-prevention stretching' classes.

The group members were soon to be sent off on their various, individual, prolonged projects and activities, around the World, and they all needed to be able to self-maintain their current 'top fitness' status for the duration of their stays. The twin swinging doors of the gym literally burst open!

"Hiiiii!!! How's everybody doing?!", cried the new arrival, camp as a row of tents and subtle as an air raid.

"Oh 'ello, 'ere we go," I thought, about the 'newby' (whom I instantly named 'Daniel'- the biblical one) - as he flounced his way in. All five feet, six inches of him, built like a starved whippet and with his arms a-waftin' like willow branches - "He's gonna get absolutely mullered!"

"Oh fuckin' hell, he'll be wantin' us tuh suck 'is cock!" mumbled one gruff (now somewhat reluctant) participant, almost inaudibly. Almost, but not completely, because Daniel, with the obvious hearing ability of a Horseshoe Bat, instantly retorted, "By the time I've finished with you dahlin', you'll be able to suck your own cock, believe you me! Right, c'mon boys'n'girls an' any others, chop-chop! Let's get started. First of all, let's see who can touch their toes without groanin'."

And with that Daniel was off, straight into it, with half the tribe of grunters reluctantly trying to follow his lead on their individual exercise mats, and the other half still standing, like human obelisks, staring at Daniel with a mix of bewilderment and shock. At which point I promptly made my excuses and left, thinking, "He's a gonner!"

Jump to the end of the week. We're in the accommodatingly large staffroom, when there's a bang on the door and in staggers Daniel, weighed down with a huge stack of chocolate boxes, cakes and bottles of booze.

"'Ere yuh go, 'elp yourselves, cos I'm not gonna 'av' 'em. Take me a year to shift that lot off me 'ips!", he cried.

"Blimey, you've got an absolute truckload there!", I exclaimed.

"Wait till yuh see what's outside the bloody door!" shouted Daniel, gesturing with a backwards flick of his head, "I could set up me own shop!"

The rufty-tufty, hairy-arsed, 'not having a bar of it' brigade, had all, individually and as group, been so impressed by Daniel's fitness, tuition and motivational attitude, that on their final day they had all, to a one, bought him a mountain of various cakes and goodies as a huge farewell 'thank you'! If ever there was a lesson to be had in how to win-over a hostile crowd, Daniel's was it!

CHAPTER 36

Lack of leadership

It would take a veritable biblical-sized tome of scribbling to cover the matters and manner of management, guidance and ongoing education within the world of (UK) physiotherapy. But at the time of writing, the situation leadership-wise seems akin to the inhabitants of Fraggle Rock trying to organise a moon landing.

Most serious of the problems, is that the direction of travel, profession-wise, is towards an almost exclusively 'Exercise Prescription Only' format of 'treatment' for all practitioners throughout the profession. Some NHS Hospital Physiotherapy Outpatient Departments have already enacted exactly that type of working model plan.

We are now at a point where Physiotherapy students are actually not being taught even the most basic of manual ('hands-on') therapies, such as massage or mobilisations (physical movement of limbs and joints by the physio'), and graduates are more adept at clicking mice than moving joints.

Within a generation, a large chunk of the physiotherapists' armoury (one which many would say actually defines what it is to be a 'physiotherapist') will have been lost and, as a learned barrister friend of mine recently said, "If all you now do is prescribe exercises, Nathan, then what, precisely, differentiates you as a physiotherapist from say, someone who's a gym instructor with a bit of anatomical knowledge?"

I had no effective reply…!

If you take your car to a garage for repair, it may be, that all it needs is a tiny bit of work, using a screwdriver to fix it. It may be that it needs slightly more work, using a screwdriver and some spanners to fix it. Or it may be that it needs extensive work, using all the tools in the garage to fix it. What you want, is a mechanic who has the complete knowledge, toolset and ability to know which task to perform, and the ability to do so successfully...

...the same goes for your physiotherapist!

CHAPTER 37

End notes

Actions guaranteed to thoroughly piss-off your physiotherapist (or other health care practitioner):

1. Saying, "I don't know if it's anything you did, but I haven't had any pain for a few days now!", after having been relieved of long-standing pain in a relatively short space of time!
2. Not saying 'Thank you' when they've resolved your problem - it's amazing how many, ordinarily polite people, forget to do so.
3. Taking your 'vital' cup of coffee or sandwich into the treatment room, ...and continuing to consume it!
4. Actually answering your mobile phone mid-treatment, ..and then having an extended conversation with the caller.
5. Huffing and puffing melodramatically, in order to emphasise just how much pain you're in.
6. Immediately telling your physio' you know exactly what's wrong with you and/or precisely what needs to be done to

'fix' you.

7. Immediately telling your physio' that you've had all sorts of other unsuccessful treatments and therefore, you know there's not the slightest chance they'll be able to help you. [NB: On points 6. & 7., even the nicest of physiotherapists will likely simply start to hear a voice in their head saying, "So why are you here then?"]
8. Being generally 'combative' - these days many patients arrive with, seemingly, the prime intention of simply arguing with or venting at their physio', some quite vehemently so - your physiotherapist generally, as a rule, wants to help you, not fight you.
9. Trying to take mum, dad, sister, half your extended family, your pet rabbit and 'Uncle Tom Cobbly & all' into the cubicle with you.

Obviously certain occasions warrant some semblance of this last scene, but there's a growing tendency now for people to have numerous family, friends and/or acquaintances accompany them during treatment sessions, often for no other reason than that the patient 'fancies a bit of company', or their companions 'just want to see what goes on' - some physiotherapists don't seem to mind this type of scenario, but many do, and I have to say that I'm one of the latter.

I fully concur with one of my (ordinarily quite reserved) colleagues who, on being faced with just such a situation, involving four extra, 'extended-family' individuals, trying to cram into a very small treatment room, once said (in an extremely thick Welsh accent), "We're an 'ospital yoo kno', not a bluddi social club!!!"

Finally:
'We're born, we live, we die, we're dust; what we do in the middle determines our legacy!' - Nathan Ohio 08/01/80

www.ingramcontent.com/pod-product-compliance
Lightning Source LLC
Chambersburg PA
CBHW072158290526
45794CB00004B/1557

9798852600899